Passion and Compassion

"To achieve the ambitious targets of Fast-Track and end AIDS as a public health threat by 2030, the work of the faith community will be critical. This fresh and thoughtful narrative describes the central role played by the World Council of Churches, and I look forward to continuing to working closely with the faith community on the last mile of this journey."

—Michel Sidibé, Executive Director, UNAIDS

Passion and Compassion

The Ecumenical Journey with HIV

Manoj Kurian

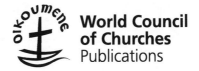

**World Council
of Churches**
Publications

PASSION AND COMPASSION
The Ecumenical Journey with HIV
Manoj Kurian

WCC Publications is the book publishing programme of the World Council of Churches. Founded in 1948, the WCC promotes Christian unity in faith, witness and service for a just and peaceful world. A global fellowship, the WCC brings together 345 Protestant, Orthodox, Anglican and other churches representing more than 550 million Christians in 110 countries and works cooperatively with the Roman Catholic Church.

Opinions expressed in WCC Publications are those of the authors.

Scripture quotations are from the New Revised Standard Version Bible, © copyright 1989 by the Division of Christian Education of the National Council of the Churches of Christ in the USA. Used by permission.

Cover design: Adele Robey
Cover image: Photo by Paul Jeffrey
Book design and typesetting: Michelle Cook / 4 Seasons Book Design
ISBN: 978-2-8254-1682-2

World Council of Churches
150 route de Ferney, P.O. Box 2100
1211 Geneva 2, Switzerland
http://publications.oikoumene.org

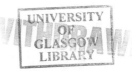

Contents

Preface

For the past 30 years, the ecumenical journey with HIV and AIDS has embodied a remarkable pilgrimage within global Christianity. In dealing with HIV, societies and faith communities not only have been challenged in the way they think and act but also have been in some measure transformed.

Since the start of the epidemic, in the 1980s, it is estimated that around 78 million people have become HIV-positive, and over 30 million people have died of AIDS and AIDS-related illnesses. Currently, nearly 37 million people globally are living with HIV. There has been rapid progress in treating HIV, and as of March 2015 over 15 million people are accessing antiretroviral therapy. Yet, only an estimated 51 percent of people with HIV know their infection status. In 2014, an estimated 2 million people became newly infected with HIV and 1.2 million people died from AIDS-related illnesses.[1]

The way the disease is transmitted[2] (sexually, mother-to-child, intravenously—including through contaminated blood and improperly sterilized medical equipment or sharing of used needles[3]), the illness' impact on people living in poverty and marginalized communities, and the suffering and stigma associated with the disease have influenced the perception of HIV and AIDS in society. This means that any successful response to HIV and AIDS has mandated the involvement of a multidimensional approach, beyond addressing the biomedical aspects of the disease.

The need for a faith response to AIDS became evident as the epidemic precipitated a crisis of enormous spiritual, social, economic, and political proportions. The impact AIDS had on the lives of individuals and communities made it essential for churches to accompany their members. People of faith responding to the crisis could well follow their foundational teachings to promote lovingkindness and compassion. But often, due to fear, ignorance, and moralistic misinterpretation of holy scripture, many faith communities stigmatized, excluded, and harmed people living with HIV. It was clear from the beginning that the church could be either part of the solution to HIV or part of the problem—or, often, both simultaneously.

The ecumenical movement has acknowledged and responded to the AIDS epidemic since 1984. It has been a journey both of suffering and of bringing succour and service to millions of people; a journey both of experiencing stigma and discrimination and of embodying the struggle for human dignity and respect. This journey has raised profound questions regarding relationships between genders in the context of patriarchy and differing power dynamics in society. It also has forced faith communities to deal with human sexuality and its diversity.

The journey has also successfully raised and coaxed responses to issues of justice and equity, with regard to access to comprehensive HIV care and support, regardless of the socioeconomic and the geographic situation of the person affected by HIV. The journey has taken us from a time of fear and despair to one of hope, discovery, solidarity, and pastoral accompaniment, expanding care and support, and significant successes in overcoming stigma and discrimination.

Apart from invoking solidarity, the journey has helped in the transformation of the church's ministry. From a predominantly charity orientation, reaching the unreached, churches and communities are increasingly approaching the vulnerable and the needy with humility and the willingness to learn from the margins of society. As the churches contribute to healing and restoration, the faith community as a whole is being healed and renewed, extending the reign of God here and now.

In helping churches and societies deal with existential challenges, bringing people together to find solutions, the ecumenical response to HIV and AIDS stands tall among other historically significant achievements of the ecumenical movement. This includes assisting with the refugee crisis in Europe after World War II and into the 1950s; the creation of worldwide ecumenical networks; the Faith and Order Commission's work on *Baptism, Eucharist and Ministry*, which has led to new worship patterns within churches; the Programme to Combat Racism, which contributed to the struggle against apartheid in South Africa; and the lifting up of the importance of interreligious dialogue and relations with other faiths as an integral part of the life of the church.[4]

This book takes you on the journey, the ecumenical pilgrimage with HIV, giving you insights into and assessing the significance of this sojourn over the last 30 years. Humanity has made great progress in dealing with HIV. With the increasing availability of treatment for HIV, the condition is increasingly becoming a chronic disease and is normalizing living with HIV. But struggles related to the relationships and life experiences of people who are vulnerable to becoming infected by HIV continue to be challenging and need to be transformed for the better. Significant proportions of the world population continue to live in fragile communities where inequities persist and where essential services do not reach the people in need. So, if HIV is seen more as a symptom of the maladies that affect our societies, success in overcoming one symptom does not always indicate victory in addressing the underlying vulnerabilities. This narrative will also help you reflect on the importance of this journey by equipping both the church and society to address the vulnerabilities we continue to face and to confront the future more successfully.

In compiling and composing this story of ecumenical engagement with HIV, I have drawn liberally from the work of my predecessors, colleagues, and collaborators in the World Council of Churches and from the many programmatic documents they have published or archived over the years. I am grateful to them and gratified that we can highlight their work in this decades-long story of engagement. I wish also to acknowledge with gratitude the many persons— interviewees, resource persons, and others who have been helpful in crafting this story—for their recollections, insights and life stories. I wish especially to extend sincere thanks Ms. Ayoko Bahun-Wilson, Dr Erlinda Senturias, Prof. Ezra Chitando, Dr. Gert Rüppell, Hendrew Lusey-Gekawaku, Prof. Dr Isabel Apawo Phiri, the Rev. Fr J. P. Mokgethi-Heath, Prof. Dr Musa Dube, Rev. Dr Nyambura Njoroge, Rev. Pauline Wanjiru Njiru, Rev. Philip Kuruvilla, and Dr Sue Parry, as well as to WCC publisher Michael West, for contributing texts and for going through the book meticulously and giving suggestions and making improvements. I am also grateful to Rev. Dr Nyambura Njoroge, the WCC's programme executive for EHAIA, for commissioning me to write this account and for our many years of work together.

I dedicate this book to all who have given their lives to equipping faith communities to face and overcome HIV.

Chapter 1

Connectedness and Accountability: The Role of the Churches

"Bear one another's burdens, and in this way,
you will fulfill the law of Christ." — Gal. 6:2

I t is indeed unique in the global religious contexts, and particularly the Christian milieu, that the ecumenical movement addressed a disease such as HIV and AIDS in a forthright and balanced manner from the earliest days of the epidemic. The ability to respond was due to the very nature of the ecumenical movement: its accountability to the needs and the suffering of member churches and their congregations; its accountability to the wider international community; its capacity to process complex issues in a consultative manner; and the presence of committed and capable people to accompany the process and take specific action. The movement's mandate and willingness to connect individual and community-level experiences and challenges to the international arena and policy space have made this journey a remarkable one.

The WCC's Accountability to Its Membership and Its Convening Role

The central goal of the ecumenical movement is the visible unity of the followers of Jesus. And while "visible unity" can be understood in various ways, it necessarily involves relationships between churches.

Churches and other ecumenical partners pray, reflect, plan, and act together. As a fellowship of some 350 Anglican, Eastern and Oriental Orthodox, Old Catholic, Protestant, independent, and united churches, nurturing such relationships is a vital facet of the WCC's vocation to support the churches and the ecumenical movement in their efforts to reach visible unity. There is no doubt that today the WCC is the most representative of all the bodies that share in the one ecumenical movement. At the same time, the WCC finds itself surrounded by a polycentric network of diverse ecumenical partners, such as non-member churches, church-related organizations, and movements of Christian people at the national, regional, and global levels.

This concept of a polycentric ecumenical movement suggests new roles and attitudes for the WCC and its constitutional obligation to foster the coherence of the movement. It is increasingly evident that the Council deploys its programmatic and relational activities with full readiness and willingness to serve as a convener for the many players in the ecumenical movement. The WCC provides leadership to the many initiatives that its ecumenical partners undertake, thereby becoming an open space for dialogue and cooperation for the many ecumenical institutions and initiatives, and offering member churches and ecumenical partners opportunities to consider together responses to key issues, at key moments in history.[1]

The movement repeatedly has proven to be a dynamic and welcoming space of grace. This is a safe and dynamic space where participants can share experiences and concerns, both the successes and the challenges that their communities face in their faith contexts, common mission, fellowship, and sharing of resources. Unique challenges are brought to the attention of the fellowship, where qualified and committed staff members of the WCC facilitate the process of discussion, dialogue, and the discernment of these challenges. The participation and engagement of member churches, denominational networks, ecumenical partners—such as church-related development agencies and national and regional ecumenical organizations, associated international organizations, and civil-society organizations—provide a broad and deep spectrum of experiences to address any given challenge. The pain, suffering, and exclusion of people living with HIV and dying of AIDS—be they gay communities and Haitians living in the United States or those affected from Zaire (now the Democratic Republic of Congo) or Belgium—came to the attention of the WCC in the early 1980s.[2]

The WCC's Christian Medical Commission

The other component of the accountability framework is the WCC's relationship with international organizations. The relationship with the United Nations began, from 1946, through the specialized body of the WCC, namely the Commission of the Churches on International Affairs (CCIA).

The other area of engagement with the international community has been through the WCC's Christian Medical Commission. Since the 19th century and for over a hundred years, medical work has been one of the main focuses of Christian missionary work, the others being education and preaching the gospel. As a result, by the 1960s thousands of Christian hospitals were serving the healthcare needs of the developing world. But with the changing perception of healthcare in a rapidly evolving world, international organizations began to question the fact that more than 90 percent of the resources for the healing ministry was devoted to curative medicine. The Tübingen I and II Consultations, co-organized by the World Council of Churches (WCC), the Lutheran World Federation (LWF), and the German Institute for Medical Mission (DIFÄM), in 1964 and 1968 addressed many of these questions. These processes called for an integrated witness where medical work could be correlated with social work, nutrition, and agriculture and community development, recognizing that medical care was only a component of a diversity of disciplines, all of which were necessary to promote and maintain health. This led to the formation of the Christian Medical Commission (CMC) in 1968.[3] The CMC assisted in reorienting the churches' healthcare ministry to evolve into a more comprehensive and community-oriented service.[4] On 22 March 1974, Dr. Halfdan Mahler, director-general of the World Health Organization (WHO), called together his senior staff for a joint meeting with all five senior staff of the CMC. As a result of this meeting, a joint committee was set up to explore the possibilities of collaboration and cooperation in "matters of mutual concerns." In spite of the disparity in size, the relationship between the two organizations turned out to be exceptionally fruitful. The most significant result of the CMC/WHO relationship was the WHO's formulation, in 1975, of the principles of primary healthcare. This marked a radical shift in WHO priorities, with massive implications for healthcare systems everywhere.[5] The experience of the grassroots organizations on community health issues was channelled to the international, intergovernmental body. The churches were able to influence and give quality experiential and experimental input into a joint study process—by the WHO and UNICEF—called "Alternative approaches to meeting basic health needs of populations in developing countries." Thus began the process of demystifying healthcare, where care services were tailored to the needs of the communities with the local population being involved in the formulation of the system's policy and delivery. This led to the development of the philosophy of primary healthcare.[6]

The primary healthcare philosophy stressed an integrated approach of preventive, curative, and promotive health services both for the community and the individual. The WHO adopted this in 1977, which implied a radical shift in the organization's priorities, with global implications for decentralizing healthcare and placing greater rights and responsibilities with people in managing their own health. The churches' contribution to the evolution in the thinking about and practice of primary healthcare is a lasting contribution to public health.[7]

In the 1970s Christian communities began to train village health workers at the grassroots level. Equipped with essential drugs and simple methods, these workers were able to treat most common diseases and to promote the use of clean water and better hygienic conditions. They facilitated the introduction of small health centres that offered low-cost inpatient care, as well as prenatal and early childhood health services. In these new, decentralized healthcare systems, many mission hospitals began to play an essential role by acting as intermediaries between local village health services and the centralized state-supported hospitals.

It is in this context of an ongoing, official relationship with the WCC that the WHO asked the WCC, in 1983, to raise awareness among the churches regarding the emerging disease called AIDS. It is to be noted that earlier that year, the U.S. Centers for Disease Control and Prevention (CDC) had released a statement that "persons who may be considered at increased risk of AIDS include those with symptoms and signs suggestive of AIDS; sexual partners of AIDS patients; sexually active homosexual or bisexual men with multiple partners; Haitian entrants to the United States; present or past abusers of IV drugs; patients with haemophilia; and sexual partners of individuals at increased risk for AIDS."[8]

Committed and Capable to Accompany Churches in Facing Complex Issues

For the churches, the challenge of HIV and AIDS has involved soul searching. Their pastoral calling to minister to the sick and marginalized has drawn many Christian institutions to care for people living with AIDS. But the connections between AIDS and sexuality, and between AIDS and paternalistic structures, have made it very difficult for churches to face up to the implications of HIV transmission, not just for Christians but for the churches themselves. Principally, because of the early identification of AIDS with homosexuality, there was a lot of resistance from many member churches, and many of the staff members were reluctant to take on the issue. It took the passion and unfailing commitment of two devoted staff members to assist the WCC and accompany its executive committee in responding clearly and positively to the pain and persecution of people living with HIV and to answer the call of the World Health Organization.

Dr Cecile De Sweemer, a Belgian medical doctor with a doctorate in international health from Johns Hopkins University and with extensive experience in Asia and Africa, as the deputy director of the Christian Medical Commission at the WCC (1982–1986) took up the issue of AIDS against all the odds. She was also responsible for dealing with other significant projects, such as advocacy work related to the Chernobyl nuclear disaster, the Bhopal industrial gas tragedy, and primary healthcare in West Africa. In dealing with the contentious issue of AIDS, Dr De Sweemer had strong allies—Rev. Dr David L. Gosling, the director of Church and Society at the WCC, and Rev Dr Jean Massamba Ma Mopolo, the Executive Secretary responsible for the Family Ministries programme, who worked with her in addressing this challenging issue in a balanced and succinct manner. Dr Gosling, who was originally a nuclear physicist before ordination and with extensive interests and experience in science, ecology, and different religions, was a dynamic partner to assist in dealing with a new and unknown challenge in the form of AIDS.

Speaking of her experience with the CMC, Dr De Sweemer said, "By 1983 the first rumours of AIDS started. I had quite a number of friends in WHO, including Dr. Assaad.[9] He kept saying, 'I cannot move because none of the governments wants to talk about it, and I think they don't want to talk about it, because they are afraid of the reactions of the religious groups if they start talking about sex.'" De Sweemer added, "When this first came to light in the U.S. it was a 'homosexual problem and a Haitian problem,' and in Belgium it was an 'African' problem." Of the three staff members of the Christian Medical Commission, only De Sweemer was willing to take on the controversial topic.[10] In 1987[11] De Sweemer recollected,

> I have great admiration for Dr. Mann[12] of the WHO and for his team. I personally feel that AIDS is one of the subjects the WHO has tackled most efficiently and most effectively. They have their own limitation, . . . as an intergovernmental organisation, they can only do what the governments let them do. . . . WHO was the one who invited the WCC to involve itself officially and openly in the debate because they could not handle the many constraints that were being put on them by governments. The governments were putting on the constraints because they thought the churches were putting on constraints.[13]

The WCC's first conference on AIDS was held in Geneva in June 1984. Facing intensive challenges, the process was kept on track by the commitment and resilience of the staff members. Various consultations and discussions led to the historic consultation held in Geneva in June 1986 on "AIDS and the Church as a Healing Community." There was tremendous opposition from within the WCC and from various quarters of its constituency because of the linking of AIDS with sin and homosexuality. With this consultation, however, the dedicated and prophetic work of the team consisting of De Sweemer, David Gosling and Jean Masamba Ma Mpolo, supported by Paul Evans, and their biblically based unwillingness to retreat finally paid off.

Based on the report from the consultation, the WCC's Executive Committee meeting in Reykjavik, Iceland, in September 1986, released a statement making prophetic recommendations to churches to face AIDS with a clarity of vision and in truth. Even after 30 years, the words are deeply moving and challenging. This visionary statement set a high standard, setting the tone for the next three decades. It was made in an era when AIDS was revealed to the world as a crisis of global and devastating proportions, a context in which, as Susan Davies states, "the Church was challenged with three terrifying realities: death, sexuality and otherness."[14] This statement was a statement of faith—a fresh breath of grace to a world weighed down with fear, condemnation, and death. The statement challenged churches to re-examine the conditions that promoted the pandemic, and to become more conscious of the human implications of broken relationships and unjust structures, and of their own complacency and complicity. Significantly, the statement did not shy away from issues related to sexuality and sexual orientation.

As a result of the WCC AIDS declaration, several of the major Christian denominations were challenged and energized to move forward in dealing with AIDS.

The WCC's Executive Committee, meeting in Reykjavik, Iceland, 15–19 September 1986, recommended that:

- The AIDS crisis challenges us profoundly to be the Church in deed and in truth: to be the Church as a healing community. AIDS is heart-breaking and challenges the churches to break their own hearts, to repent of inactivity and of rigid moralisms. Since AIDS cuts across race, class, gender, age, sexual orientation and sexual expression, it challenges our fears and exclusions. The healing community itself will need to be healed by the forgiveness of Christ.

The consultation called on the churches to undertake the following:

1. Pastoral Care
   - The people of God can be the family that embraces and sustains those who are sick with AIDS or AIDS-related conditions, caring for the brother, sister or child without barriers, exclusion, hostility or rejection.

   - Death is a mystery. We are angry and helpless when faced by its reality. We need to acknowledge our helplessness and not deny it. This has particular significance as we share the experience of ministry with persons with AIDS and as we are ministered to by them, as we grow with them in a Christian understanding of death in the light of Christ's death and resurrection.

2. Education for Prevention
   - To assure high-quality information on the disease, we invite the churches to participate actively with the health professions, local governments, where possible, and local community agencies in programmes of prevention education. We invite the churches to use the World Health Organisation and its networks of local resources.

   - AIDS is preventable. Society must concentrate sufficient resources on its prevention. This will involve measures that should reasonably be adopted by all: carriers, the sick, current high-risk groups and the general population since the latter includes many undetected carriers. It also calls urgently for responsible forms of behaviour by all, and for the improvement of physical and socio-economic conditions in many parts of the world.

   - Preventive measures and altered behaviour patterns must address the different factors that favour the transmission of the virus; it is necessary, therefore, that the different modes of transmission prevalent regionally should be clearly described and understood.

3. Social Ministry
   - Given the widely varying valuations of some of the issues related to the disease, member churches and ecumenical councils will have to be rigorously contextual in their response. We affirm, however, certain commonly held values, especially:
     a. the free exchange of medical and educational information about the disease within countries and across borders;

b. the freedom to pursue research about the disease;

c. the free flow of information about the disease to patients, their families and loved ones;

d. the right to medical and pastoral care regardless of socio-economic status, race, sex, sexual orientation or sexual relationships;

e. the privacy of medical records of persons with AIDS or AIDS-related Complex or positive antibodies.

- Since AIDS is a global epidemic, effective action by churches and individual Christians must extend not only to the AIDS neighbour closest at hand but also through effective global collaboration to the stranger on the farthest side of the world.

The consultation also called on the churches "to work against the real danger that AIDS will be used as an excuse for discrimination and oppression and to work to ensure the protection of the human rights of persons affected directly or indirectly by AIDS."

The Executive Committee also wishes to call to the attention of the churches these further concerns expressed by the consultation:

- to confess that churches as institutions have been slow to speak and to act, that many Christians have been quick to judge and condemn many of the people who have fallen prey to the disease; and that through their silence, many churches share responsibility for the fear that has swept our world more quickly than the virus itself.

- to affirm and support the entire medical and research community in its efforts to combat the disease.

- to affirm that God deals with us in love and mercy and that we are therefore freed from simplistic moralizing about those who are attacked by the virus.

The Response and Periodic Follow-Up

Through the 30-year journey, critical consultations on the issue were held at regular intervals, to assess the churches' response to HIV and AIDS, to issue guidance, and to mobilize support to churches to adapt and bring coherence to their responses.

As the spread of HIV infection and AIDS continued at a relentless and frightening pace, by the end of 1996 the estimated number of people living with

HIV was 23 million. With just one antiretroviral drug, zidovudine (AZT), available as a treatment for HIV, which was not widely available and against which drug resistance was rapidly developing, and with AIDS testing kits not easily available, the fear and the stigma associated with HIV spread even faster.

As a response of the call from the ecumenical movement in 1986, the WCC developed and distributed widely key educational and pastoral resources in multiple languages, promoting awareness regarding HIV and AIDS in the context of faith communities. The three popular key resources were *What Is AIDS? A Manual for Health Workers* (1987), and *Learning about HIV and AIDS: A Manual for Pastors and Teachers* (1989, with later revised editions published in 1994, 2002, and 2006), both written by Dr. Birgitta Rubenson, and *A Guide to HIV/AIDS Pastoral Counselling* (1990), edited by Rev. Jorge Maldonado, with support from the AIDS Working Group guided by WCC Executive Secretary Dr Erlinda Senturias, who coordinated the HIV and AIDS Program from 1989 to 1997. Dr Senturias, together with Ms. Yvonne Kambale Kavuo, coordinated the participatory action research on AIDS and the community as a source of care and healing in Uganda, Tanzania, and Zaire from 1991 to 1993. The result of the research was reported at the WCC Central Committee meeting in Johannesburg in January 1994.

In Africa, encouraged by the WCC, the Tanzanian, Ugandan, and Democratic Republic of Congo (DRC, then Zaire) Protestant medical agencies set up an experimental Participatory Action Research (PAR) programme. PAR enabled communities to do their own research, identify the issues that needed to be addressed, and develop strategies for dealing with those issues. This system was succinctly described and presented in a handbook called *Confronting AIDS Together: Participatory Methods in Addressing the HIV/AIDS Epidemic.*[15]

Women and HIV

Even at the onset of the AIDS epidemic, when the crisis was overwhelmingly perceived as primarily concerning homosexual communities, staff at the WCC lifted up the vulnerability of women.[16] To correspond with the fourth World Conference on Women, held in Beijing in 1995, the WCC drew together experiences of women's health and the challenge of HIV from Brazil, Argentina, Costa Rica, Chile, India, Thailand, Papua New Guinea, Uganda, DRC (Zaire), Tanzania, and the USA. The consultation was held in India because China refused entry to people with HIV. It revealed the fact that attitudes to women were (and still are) so ingrained in the cultures of communities that, for most of the world's population, it was almost impossible for individuals to change their behaviour except in the context of a general decision within the community, where such transformation must occur. These further challenged churches to advocate for policy changes that make women less vulnerable to being affected by HIV. The findings of this programme, and the stories of many of the people who took part in it, appear in Gillian Paterson's *Love in a Time of AIDS*.[17] The topic was also addressed comprehensively in an issue of *Contact*, titled "Women and AIDS: Building Healing Communities."[18] (*Contact* is a publication focussed on the health-related work of the World Council of Churches, being published since 1970).

Consolidating an Ecumenical Policy on HIV and AIDS

Deeply concerned about the rapidly unfolding epidemic, in 1994 the WCC Central Committee meeting in Johannesburg, South Africa, mandated the formation of a consultative group to conduct a study on HIV and AIDS. The group, headed by Dr Christoph Benn, of the DIFÄM, consisted of medical and nonmedical professionals, clergy, religious and laypersons, all of them either living with or working with HIV and AIDS. They were charged with looking into the pastoral, ethical, human rights, prevention, care, and support issues of people living with HIV and AIDS, as well as related matters of human rights and justice. When the two-year process began, the group set out with apparently irreconcilable differences of approaches. But, during the process, the members of the consultative group experienced a high degree of convergence and common vision. Members describe a sense of unity and inspiration in listening to each other, in worshipping together, and in the various encounters with the reality of HIV and AIDS in different cultural contexts. The process became a good example for the difficult task of combining the disciplines of systematic theology, pastoral care, and sexual and moral ethics to formulate principles to help Christians and churches worldwide in developing their own strategies to respond to the AIDS epidemic.[19]

The landmark result of the global study was reported to the WCC Central Committee in 1996, which in turn adopted a statement based on the WCC consultative group on AIDS study process and report, in September 1996. The results of the study were also published in various languages as a WCC study document, *Facing AIDS: The Challenge, the Churches' Response,* in 1997.[20] The study elaborated clear policy guidelines for the churches to implement in order to face the challenge of HIV and AIDS effectively and in an inclusive manner.

WCC Study Document: *Facing AIDS: The Challenge, the Churches' Response* (1997)

Conclusion: What can the churches do?

Points for common reflection and action by the churches:

A. *The life of the churches: responses to the challenge of HIV/AIDS*

1. We ask the churches to provide a climate of love, acceptance and support for those who are vulnerable to, or affected by, HIV/AIDS.

2. We ask the churches to reflect together on the theological basis for their response to the challenges posed by HIV/AIDS.

3. We ask the churches to reflect together on the ethical issues raised by the pandemic, interpret them in their local context and to offer guidance to those confronted by difficult choices.

4. We ask the churches to participate in the discussion in society at large of ethical issues posed by HIV/AIDS, and to support their own members who, as health care professionals, face difficult ethical choices in the areas of prevention and care.

B. *The witness of the churches in relation to immediate effects and causes of HIV/AIDS*

1. We ask the churches to work for better care for persons affected by HIV/AIDS.

2. We ask the churches to give particular attention to the conditions of infants and children affected by the HIV/AIDS pandemic and to seek ways to build a supportive environment.

3. We ask the churches to help safeguard the rights of persons affected by HIV/AIDS and to study, develop and promote the human rights of people living with HIV/AIDS through mechanisms at national and international levels.

4. We ask the churches to promote the sharing of accurate information about HIV/AIDS, to promote a climate of open discussion and to work against the spread of misinformation and fear.

5. We ask the churches to advocate increased spending by governments and medical facilities to find solutions to the problems—both medical and social—raised by the pandemic.

C. *The witness of the churches in relation to long-term causes and factors encouraging the spread of HIV/AIDS*

1. We ask the churches to recognize the linkage between AIDS and poverty, and to advocate measures to promote just and sustainable development.

2. We urge that special attention be focussed on situations that increase the vulnerability to AIDS such as migrant labour, mass refugee movements and commercial sex activity.

3. In particular, we ask the churches to work with women as they seek to attain the full measure of their dignity and express the full range of their gifts.

4. We ask the churches to educate and involve youth and men in order to prevent the spread of HIV/AIDS.

5. We ask the churches to seek to understand more fully the gift of human sexuality in the contexts of personal responsibility, relationships, family and Christian faith.

6. We ask the churches to address the pandemic of drug use and the role this plays in the spread of HIV/AIDS and to develop locally relevant responses in terms of care, de-addiction, rehabilitation and prevention.

The study places the onus of response to AIDS on the churches. The very relevance of faith communities is manifested by their reflection, openness, contextual interpretations, and provision of an enabling environment for the AIDS response. The churches and Christians are challenged to be empathetic, compassionate, and helpful, to protect the rights and dignity of the vulnerable, and to advocate for treatment and care in the wider society. The study also marks a dramatic and notable shift of emphasis from "personal sin" (which was the dominant interpretation) to "structural sin" in the context of HIV and AIDS. The study lifts up the responsibility of churches and faith communities to work at reducing the vulnerability of marginalized sections of the populations to the effects of HIV and AIDS, implying the sin of not doing the right thing. Here, the ecumenical movement demonstrated creativity and leadership in a context where older notions of sin were prevalent.

One of the important aspects linked to the study was the insight that fact finding and presentation have to go along with information, enlightenment, and education. This insight led to the collaborative work of the CMC–HIV

Study Programme, led by Dr Senturias of the WCC, and the WCC Education in Mission desk, headed by Dr Gert Rüppell, in developing a manual to accompany the study. Two factors were decisive in the production of this manual. First, the meeting of the consultative group on HIV and AIDS in Delhi, India, in February 1996, where a special group of educators focussed on transforming the study insights into educational materials. The second factor was the vital contributions made through the group's cooperation with the Evangelical Lutheran Church of Chile's Program for Health Education (EPES), focussing on HIV and AIDS-related work, which ensured that the education material was accessible and illustrated. The final version of the manual *Facing Aids: Education in the Context of Vulnerability*, identified as "Study Guide Accompanying the World Council of Churches' Study Document on HIV/AIDS,"[21] was produced in three languages (English, Spanish, and French) in collaboration between the WCC and the EPES in Santiago, Chile, under the leadership of Karen Anderson (EPES) and Gert Rüppell (Unit II/WCC). The study material contains a structured framework for group learning sessions, designed to equip resource group leaders to undertake HIV and AIDS awareness building. It has been a very popular and effective tool for the enlightenment of pastors and congregations in dealing with HIV.

Responding to the Call of Churches from Africa

Most of the available epidemiological data indicate that the extensive spread of HIV started in sub-Saharan Africa in the late 1970s. By the early 1980s, HIV was found in a geographic band stretching from West Africa across to the Indian Ocean; the countries north of the Sahara and those in the southern cone of the continent remained apparently untouched. By 1987, the epidemic began gradually to move south.[22]

In 1987, De Sweemwer, who worked for CMC-WCC, said, "Africa has to act now. And that was my undivided advice, for example, to the Minister of Health in Nigeria, Prof Ransome-Kuti, an old colleague of mine with whom, for the past 20 years, I have been struggling to build up primary healthcare in Nigeria. My reason is that AIDS is different from most of the other conditions in that it has a long latency time. It is a time bomb where waiting means that the problem will increase, where not informing the population means that the problem will increase, and basically the people will become victims of their own lack of knowledge. . . ."[23]

By 1998, sub-Saharan Africa was home to 70 percent of the 5.8 million people who became infected with HIV. It is also the region in which four-fifths of all the 2.5 million AIDS deaths occurred in 1998. It was the global epicentre, continuing to dwarf the rest of the world on the AIDS balance sheet, though only a tenth of the world's population lived in the region. The sheer number of people affected by the epidemic in sub-Saharan Africa was overwhelming. AIDS being responsible for an estimated 2 million African deaths that year meant 5,500 funerals a day. And, despite the scale of death, there were 21.5 million adults and a further 1 million children living with HIV. While no country in Africa had escaped the virus, countries in the East and especially in Southern Africa were more severely affected than others. Societies and churches were para-lyzed.[24] Villages and schools were empty and farms were lying fallow. But even in that devastating situation, women in the churches started home-based care by attending to the sick and dying as part of their service.[25]

At the eighth WCC General Assembly in Harare, Zimbabwe, in 1998, there was a clear call from Christians and churches in Africa to the global fellowship of churches to journey with them in overcoming the overwhelming HIV pandemic. As a response, following the assembly, the Health and Healing programme of the WCC conducted several regional consultations on HIV and AIDS, with church leaders and ecumenical partners, including, notably, in East Africa, in January 2001, in Mukono-Kampala, Uganda (in collaboration with All Africa Conference of Churches); in Southern Africa, in March 2001, in Johannesburg (in collaboration with South African Council of Churches); and in West Africa, in April 2001, in Dakar, Senegal (in collaboration with All Africa Conference of Churches and Medical Assistance Programme [MAP] International). The series concluded with the "Global Consultation on the Ecumenical Response to the Challenge of HIV/AIDS in Africa," held in Nairobi, Kenya, 25–28 November 2001. The consultation involved three groups of partners: churches, ecumeni-cal groups, and church-related organizations in Africa; churches, ecumenical groups, and church-related organizations in Europe and North America; and the World Council of Churches. The consultation clearly identified stigma and discrimination as a fundamental impediment to overcoming HIV. The global gathering condemned discrimination and stigmatization of people living with HIV and AIDS as a sin and contrary to the will of God.

The consultation produced a paradigm shift in the ecumenical response to HIV and led to a visionary and groundbreaking "Plan of Action" (2001) on ecumenical HIV response, with commitments that later paved the way for the launching and implementation of the Ecumenical HIV and AIDS Initiative in Africa (EHAIA) by the WCC in 2002. The Plan of Action identified HIV and

AIDS as major threats to dignity, human development, social cohesion, political stability, and as devastating to the economic sustainability of families and society at large in sub-Saharan countries. The consultation also highlighted harmful cultural practices and theological and ethical fault lines in the practice of ministry in the churches and theological institutions. The initiative also launched a global effort to stimulate theological and ethical reflection, dialogue, and exchange on issues related to HIV and AIDS.

In 2001, the WCC joined forces with the Christian medical relief organiation MAP International–Eastern Africa, under the leadership of Dr Peter Okaalet, to conduct two consultations in Kenya sponsored by the Joint United Nations Programme on HIV/AIDS (UNAIDS), on HIV and theological education. In 2002, based on the input received from the two consultations from academic deans, principals, and theologians of various denominations from 20 theological institutions in 14 countries, the WCC, under the leadership of Dr Musa Dube, fully revised and published a new "HIV and AIDS Curriculum for Theological Institutions in Africa,"[26] based on a first version of a curriculum published by MAP. This work eventually progressed to be developed into WCC-initiated Theological Education by Extension Modules, in the context of HIV.

After the Nairobi consultation, the Ecumenical HIV and AIDS Initiative in Africa (EHAIA) was created and launched to provide a service—to sharpen skills, to break the silence and shame, and to bring down barriers of discrimination and stigma that divided the community—so that churches would be transformed to channel hope and life in its fullness. WCC-EHAIA's two-pronged approach involved promoting HIV competence among churches in Africa and working with theological institutions to integrate and mainstream HIV into theological curricula. Ecumenical partners such as the Brot für die Welt, ICCO, Norwegian Church AIDS, Christian AID, Hilfswerk der Evangelischen Kirchen Schweiz, Evangelical Lutheran Church in America, and many others have played a crucial role in ensuring that this initiative is funded and engaged and present on the ground.

Until 2006, WCC-EHAIA was housed in the WCC Health and Healing programme, but following the WCC General Assembly in Porto Alegre, Brazil, it became a separate entity under the Justice and Peace work of the WCC. Christoph Mann, with great sincerity and in a systematic manner, helped establish the initiative and served as the first project coordinator of WCC-EHAIA (2002–2007). He was followed by Rev. Dr Nyambura Njoroge in 2007, and at the time of writing this book she continues to guide WCC-EHAIA with passion and dedication. WCC-EHAIA has been guided by an International Reference Group (IRG), consisting of church leaders, religious leaders living with HIV, ecumenical partners, and technical experts from international organizations. Musa W. Dube was the theology consultant to WCC-EHAIA from 2002 to 2004. She played a major role in mobilizing theological institutions to transform their curricula to address HIV and AIDS. Her role was effectively taken over by Professor Ezra Chitando (2004 to date) and Rev. Charles Kaagba (2004–2015). WCC-EHAIA was always close to the churches and people in the different regions, attentive to the needs of churches in the AIDS response and accompanying them in their journey to be competent and compassionate. The regional work has been guided successfully by regional coordinators and their regional staff. These include Dr Sue Parry (2002–2014) in Southern Africa, Hendrew Lusey-Gekawaku (2002 to date) in Central Africa, Ayoko Bahun-Wilson in West Africa (2003 to date), Ms. Jacinta Maingi (2002–2008) and Rev. Pauline Wanjiru Njiru (2009 to date) in East Africa, and Rev. Deolinda Dorcas Teca (2007–2012) and Rev. Dr Luciano Chanhelela Chianeque (2012 to date) for Lusophone Africa. WCC-EHAIA has greatly benefitted from the conscientious contributions of the administrative staff based at the WCC, namely, Ms. Tania Zarraga (2002–2008) and Ms. Lona Lupali (2008 to date).

The churches and people of Africa are the wellspring of hope to the world in facing HIV, bringing faith, courage, innovation, and expertise. At the tenth WCC General Assembly, held in Busan, South Korea, in 2013, WCC-EHAIA was given the mandate to expand beyond Africa, to begin in Jamaica, Philippines, and Ukraine, countries where churches have reached out and requested that WCC-EHAIA share its experience and expertise from Africa. The name was therefore changed in 2014 to Ecumenical HIV and AIDS Initiatives and Advocacy, thus retaining the WCC-EHAIA acronym.

International Commitments and Outreach

Continuing and building on the relationship of the WCC with the WHO, a working relationship was developed with UNAIDS, formed in 1996. In 1999, with the financial support of UNAIDS and the guidance of Ms. Aurorita Mendoza (the person in UNAIDS responsible for gender issues and faith-based organizations at that time), the WCC's education module *Facing AIDS: Education in the Context of Vulnerability*[27] was implemented in five countries in Africa and Asia.

The WCC and its partners also participated actively in the first major AIDS conference held outside Europe and North America in July 2000, in Durban, South Africa. This conference highlighted the problems sub-Saharan Africa and other low-income countries face in tackling the HIV and AIDS epidemic. This was immediately followed by the UN Security Council passing a resolution recognizing the threat HIV and AIDS poses to international and regional stability, and a call for further action on HIV and AIDS prevention and care went out to all member states (U.N.S.C, 2000). This was reiterated at the Millennium Summit in September 2000, where the UN General Assembly voted to have an emergency special session to tackle the HIV and AIDS problem (G.A. Resolution, 2000). Following the Millennium Summit, with only nine months of preparation time, UNAIDS organized the UN General Assembly Special Session on HIV and AIDS (UNGASS), held in June 2001. This was the first conference dedicated exclusively to HIV and AIDS and also the first UN conference to explicitly involve civil-society groups in the entire process.[28]

The WCC participated in UNGASS 2001. Dr Christoph Benn led a plenary presentation, stating that the church's commitment to work cooperatively with all people living with HIV and AIDS and with people of other religious communities, community-based organizations, governments, and UN agencies in responding to HIV and AIDS. He offered the resources the churches have in the community: their local community presence, influence, the spirit of volunteerism, and genuine compassion facilitated by their spiritual mandate. He reiterated that governments alone could not achieve the goals set out but would have to coordinate with UN organizations, civil society, and NGOs, including faith-based organizations, to tackle the HIV and AIDS problem effectively and decisively.[29]

When WCC-EHAIA was formed in 2002, UNAIDS nominated Mr Calle Almedal as an advisor to the initiative and as a member of the International Reference Group. He gave critical input to WCC-EHAIA and the wider ecumenical and Catholic HIV interventions. Mr Almedal was the first person to promote the concept of "HIV-competent faith communities." He felt that faith communities were doing well in "outreach" in responding to the challenges posed by HIV in communities. But he challenged churches and faith communities to reflect deeply on the HIV and to invest in "in-reach," to transform the hearts and minds of the congregations. UNAIDS, with the guidance of Mr Almedal, was instrumental in organizing a global theological workshop focusing on HIV- and AIDS-related stigma, in Windhoek, Namibia (2003).[30] The consultation offered an effective framework for theological reflection to deal with HIV- and AIDS-related stigma. Almedal also encouraged WCC-EHAIA to engage more intentionally and creatively with the theme of human sexuality in the context of HIV and AIDS.

In that tradition, Ms. Sally Smith, the UNAIDS adviser on faith-based organizations at the time of this writing, continues to provide crucial leadership within the UN family, bringing greater collaboration and synergy with faith organizations and communities. Ms. Smith is a member of the strategy group that advises the WCC-Ecumenical Advocacy Alliance (WCC-EAA).

Mobilizing Churches across the World

In 2000, the WCC along with its ecumenical partners, initiated the Ecumenical Advocacy Alliance (EAA) as an international network of churches and church-related organizations committed to campaigning together on common concerns. The ecumenical partners chose HIV and AIDS as one of the two pressing issues around which to do global advocacy. HIV remains one of the two campaigns to date. The Global Campaign on HIV, called "Live the Promise," facilitates fighting stigma and discrimination, promoting prevention, mobilizing resources, advocating universal access to treatment, and promoting accountability of governments and churches. The Alliance equips and ensures that churches have the much-needed capacity to undertake this advocacy. Linda Hartke, the first executive director of the EAA (2000–2009), and later Peter Prove (2010–2014) with the support of the EAA team—communications officer Sara Speicher, and campaign coordinators Thabo Sephuma (2006–2009), Ruth Foley (2009–2013), and currently Francesca Merico (2015 to date)—and the strategy group focusing on the HIV campaign, ensured the global convergence of the campaign, bringing the different denominations and participants together as a recognizable force in international advocacy on HIV. Since 2004, the EAA has coordinated faith-based events at every International AIDS Conference, including ecumenical and interfaith pre-conferences. At UN meetings, particularly at High-Level Meetings, the EAA has organized joint events, including an interfaith prayer breakfast at the 2011 High-Level Meetings in collaboration with UN agencies and other faith-based organizations. WCC hosted the EAA administratively for the first seven years of its existence. After a stint as an independent organization from 2008 to 2014, the EAA was reorganized as an ecumenical initiative within the WCC. The Alliance's most recent efforts on HIV and AIDS have focused on access to treatment and advocacy to overcome stigma and discrimination, particularly through dialogue between religious leaders and people living with HIV.

Key commitments were taken by churches, facilitated by ecumenical organizations, spurring them to action in all regions of the world, making significant progress in establishing initiatives, and providing practical support on the ground. This global response found their voices at ecumenical gatherings of: Asian churches at Chiang Mai, Thailand, in November 2001, and in Colombo,

Sri Lanka, in July 2002; churches and ecumenical organizations of Eastern Europe and Central Asia in St. Petersburg, Russia, in December 2002; churches of Africa in Yaoundé, Cameroon, in November 2003; churches in the Pacific in Nandi, Fiji, in April 2004;[31] a regional meeting, "The Church and HIV/AIDS in Latin America and the Caribbean," facilitated by the Latin American Council of Churches (CLAI) and WCC in Panama City, Panama, in February 2004;[32] churches and church-related organizations of Latin America, in Quito, Ecuador, in December 2004;[33] and the churches in the Caribbean, in Georgetown, Guyana, in January 2005.[34]

The WCC Central Committee, meeting on 6 September 2006, in Geneva, reviewed the work of the ecumenical movement and recommitted the churches to become more compassionate and competent in the response to HIV and AIDS. The Central Committee also exhorted the faith-based communities to take up their responsibility to advocate for antiretroviral treatments as well as treatment for other opportunistic infections to be made available and accessible to all. The leaders of the churches were encouraged to exercise their role as advocates for just policies and to hold governments accountable for their promises.[35]

Breaking the Silence across Denominations

The first decade of the 20th century saw a great awakening of churches, denominational networks, church-related networks and development partners, and interreligious networks. They gathered, reflected, made statements at the highest level, and formulated commitments and plans to act, thereby breaking the silence on HIV and AIDS, working against stigma and discrimination, and committing to care and accompaniment.

In the year 2001 the Church of Norway Bishops Conference, the Southern African Catholic Bishops Conference, and the Anglican Communion across Africa took a prophetic stand on HIV. The latter group called their plan "Our Vision, Our Hope: The First Step."[36] In 2002 the Pan-African Lutheran Church Leadership, the Lutheran World Federation (LWF), the Anglican primates on HIV/AIDS (Canterbury), the Council of Anglican Provinces in Africa (CAPA), and the World YWCA committed to breaking the silence on HIV.

The year 2003 saw myriad responses to the HIV and AIDS crisis across denominations. The Lutheran World Federation's Latin America region developed a plan of action for "Compassion, Conversion, Care," and in the same year, at their tenth assembly in Winnipeg, Canada, the LWF took a public and prophetic stand on removing barriers that exclude people living with HIV. In the same year, the Anglican primates sent a pastoral letter to the entire Anglican Communion on HIV and AIDS, declaring that the "Body of Christ has AIDS." The letter asserted, "AIDS is not a punishment from God, for God does not visit disease and death upon his people," and went on to say, "it is rather an effect of fallen creation and our broken humanity."[37]

Also in 2003, the global network of Protestant churches, known as the Council for World Mission, also committed to becoming more caring, welcoming, and healing communities that would no longer stigmatize, exclude, and discriminate against our brothers and sisters living with HIV and AIDS. The World YWCA made a World Council Resolution that addressed HIV from the perspective of reproductive health and sexuality. Norwegian Church Aid acknowledged that HIV and AIDS had hindered development at all levels and committed, as an organization, to work to overcome stigma, promote prevention, care and support, and advocate for transformation.

The Symposium of Episcopal Conference of Africa and Madagascar (S.E.C.A.M) declared solidarity with brothers and sisters living with HIV and AIDS. They identified those affected and living with HIV as part of the body of Christ (1 Cor. 12:12) and committed to making available the church's resources, including educational and healthcare institutions and social services, to the AIDS response.

The East Central Africa Division of the Seventh-day Adventist Church committed to ensuring the rights, dignity, care, and support for people living with and affected by HIV/AIDS. They also committed to fundraising for prevention and care and support programmes in the local churches and communities. The Church of Nigeria (Anglican Communion) declared itself as a caring church in a hurting world and established policy guidelines for the national church response to HIV and AIDS.

In Asia, the Catholic Bishops of Myanmar and Catholic Bishops of India sent pastoral letters on HIV and AIDS to their national constituencies, guiding them to respond as followers of Christ. Asian Church Leadership, coming under the umbrella of the Lutheran World Federation and the United Evangelical Mission, also committed to the AIDS response, calling it the "Covenant of Life" in Indonesia.

In 2004 the Patriarch of the Romanian Orthodox Church, His Beatitude Teoctist, in his message urged love and tolerance for those suffering from AIDS and HIV. In the same year, the World Alliance of YMCA developed Global Capacity Building Forums on HIV and AIDS and a Strategic Framework for a Global YMCA Action Plan on HIV and AIDS.

Also in 2004, the United Methodist Church (UMC) resolved to establish "The United Methodist Global AIDS Fund" to raise resources to assist local congregations and conferences in identifying and creating global partnerships for mutual HIV and AIDS ministry. In the same year, the UMC highlighted the connection between alcohol, drugs, and HIV and AIDS, urging the Office of the Special Program on Substance Abuse and Related Violence (SPSARV) of the General Board of Global Ministries and all boards and agencies of the denomination to work cooperatively on issues related to drugs and AIDS.

In the same year, the United Evangelical Mission (UEM), in its HIV/AIDS Programme Policy, adopted by UEM's general assembly in Manila, looked at HIV from a theological frame, reaffirming the role of the church as a healing community, and frankly addressing human sexuality and human dignity.

In 2002, the African Network of Religious Leaders Living with and Personally Affected by HIV and AIDS (ANERELA+) was formed by the group of inspired leaders that included Rev. Canon Gideon Byamugisha, the Rev. Fr J. P. Mokgethi-Heath, Rev. Christo Greyling, and Rev. Phumzile Mabizela. The movement has since spread to other regions and in 2006 evolved into INERELA+ (International Network of Religious Leaders—lay and ordained, women and men—Living with, or Personally Affected by, HIV). The ecumenical movement, WCC-EHAIA and many church-related organizations such as Christian AID and World Vision have been accompanying this vital movement through its journey of service. The leadership of ANERELA+ and later INERELA+ have also been torchbearers in the ecumenical journey with HIV and AIDS and have been vital in breaking the silence on HIV within the churches and other faith communities.

Ecumenical work catalyzing national and international church-related AIDS movements

In countries such as Germany, Sweden, Norway, the Netherlands, the United Kingdom, and the United States of America, the churches have played a crucial role in combating HIV and AIDS both nationally and internationally. Their ecumenical commitment and engagement have been a catalyst for contributions to combating HIV and AIDS. One example is Germany. The churches in Germany and related organizations such as Brot für die Welt ("Bread for the World") have had strong partnership with churches, communities, and civil society in different regions in the world, including sub-Saharan Africa. So, with the onset of the AIDS epidemic, in solidarity with their partners, the churches' engagement with HIV and AIDS began at a very early stage, be it in South Africa, Kenya, Tanzania, or the Democratic Republic of Congo. Simultaneously, the churches in Germany began engaging with HIV both at the level of the congregation and nationally. In 1994, the first AIDS pastoral-care centre in Hamburg opened, sponsored by the local church district of the North Elbian Evangelical Lutheran Church (Nordelbische Evangelisch-Lutherische Kirche [NEK]),[38] and the Evangelical Church in Württemberg began providing AIDS pastoral care with study days, worship services, and help provided by church-appointed AIDS counsellors.

Support for these projects is provided by representatives of the AIDS working group of the Deutsches Institut für Ärztliche Mission (DIFÄM; "German Institute for Medical Mission"), which acts as a national centre of health expertise for German Protestant aid agencies. The group was founded in 2001 upon the recommendation of the Evangelische Kirche in Deutschland (EKD) Council (Evangelical Church in Germany, a body of 20 Lutheran, Reformed, and United Churches). Brot für die Welt has also appointed additional advisors to work on HIV and AIDS.[39]

The continued solidarity and partnerships ensured that the churches and organizations in Germany had a finger on the pulse of the communities affected by HIV in different regions. They were quick to discern positive movements, support ecumenical initiatives, and encourage the sharing of lessons, by lifting up best practices and positive leadership and cutting down duplication of efforts. The international ecumenical engagement further enriched the experience and influence of the churches and ecumenical organization in Germany both nationally and abroad. An example of this is the creation of "Action against AIDS" (Aktionsbündnis gegen AIDS), which was founded in Germany in 2002, inspired by the Ecumenical Advocacy Alliance. Since 2002, Action against AIDS Germany advocates with the German government to meet its responsibilities as an economically privileged country by making an appropriate contribution to the global fight against HIV and AIDS. In particular, this implies the provision of universal access to HIV prevention, treatment, care, and support to all people—especially in disadvantaged regions of the world. Action against AIDS Germany has grown to become a nationwide network of about 300 groups and organizations, local AIDS assistance groups, Protestant and Catholic churches and communities, as well as organizations working in the field of development cooperation, humanitarian aid, HIV and AIDS, and health issues. They mobilize public opinion in Germany to lobby national and international political decision makers to make greater allocation of resources for fighting AIDS.[40]

The Core Attitude of Accountability

The connectedness, inclusivity, and responsiveness to the pain and joys of the people in communities and the possibility of converging their voices to affect change globally has been a unique strength of the ecumenical movement. But this strength will only remain if the movement remains accountable to the foundational values of Christianity, to its membership, and to the wider international community.

Rev. Dr Olav Fykse Tveit, general secretary of the World Council of Churches, speaking at the "Religious Leadership in Response to HIV: A Summit of High Level Religious Leaders," in Amsterdam, in March 2010, addressed the other global religious leaders as "fellow travellers on the journey of faith." He pointed out that "the core attitude of accountability is appropriate when we talk about the past, but also what shall bring us forward together; to give quality to the formation of cultures and our relationships. If anything, what we are here to discuss and improve are our human relationships—in so many dimensions."[41]

In the case of HIV and AIDS, the ecumenical movement has provided the effective platform for interchurch collaboration, a dynamic environment for discussion, dialogue, and joint action, in order to bring about change both in the local community and the international arena. The ecumenical movement has brought out the prophetic voices and set high standards, in a very public manner, as demanded by Christ's teachings in the face of a crisis such as AIDS, for denominations and Christian communities to face the pandemic with a reflective and contrite heart.

Chapter 2

Back to Basics: The Teaching of Jesus Christ in the Context of HIV

The church, from its earliest days, defined its ministry and mission as one that offers wholistic, life-giving healing in response to people's diverse needs. Indeed, a significant factor in the growth of the early church was the fact that it presented itself as a healing movement and agent in the societies within which it took root with the gospel. Its distinctive attitude to the sick, the weak, and the vulnerable set it apart and found expression particularly through the monastic movement. Through wars, epidemics, and all the vicissitudes of human life, Christianity across the centuries has been marked by its commitment to healing ministry, which has taken many different forms.[1] The Athens conference of the Commission on World Mission and Evangelism (CWME), held in 2005, paid special attention to the church's call to be a healing community. As one of its preparatory papers affirmed: "It belongs to the very essence of the church—understood as the body of Christ created by the Holy Spirit—to live as a healing community, to recognize and nurture healing charisms and to maintain ministries of healing as visible signs of the presence of the kingdom of God."[2]

In the early days of the epidemic, the diagnosis of HIV was synonymous with marginalization, stigma, fear, and death. With the high prevalence of HIV among gays and intravenous-drug users from the onset of the epidemic, many religious individuals and churches approached HIV with moralistic judgment against persons related to their lifestyles, sexual practices, and sexual orientation. But in so doing, they betrayed the call to the church and Christian communities to live as a healing community. In this context of fear, bigotry, and deeply damaging misinterpretation of scripture, HIV has forced us to unpack Christ's teaching to its basics. The ecumenical movement has played a key role in this process. This chapter analyzes the deep motivations and transformative thinking that have made the 30-year ecumenical journey with HIV and AIDS possible for churches. It shows how the teaching of Jesus Christ helps us to address HIV and AIDS in a forthright manner and enlightens us to reflect on the vulnerabilities and complexities of societies that leave us all affected by HIV and AIDS.

The Two Faces

Even though faith communities have delivered much of the care and accompaniment for the people living with AIDS in their vicinity, many of the people living with AIDS have not felt welcome among congregations, and are often excluded or even persecuted. Faith communities have contributed to the moralistic stigmatization and discrimination that HIV-positive persons and their loved ones already face in health facilities, schools, the workplace, local communities, and in families.

Social stigma refers to any attribute that marks the bearer as culturally inferior or unacceptable. Discrimination is stigma acted upon. The association of a disease with an already stigmatized group or groups serves to divide the world of AIDS into "us" and "them," with "them" conceived as individuals at risk of infection and all associated with those individuals.[3] Stigma serves to reinforce social norms by defining deviance and demarcating "them" from "us." "Us" is more of a theoretical situation where the faith community tries to place itself on a high moral pedestal. This is reinforced by attempts to imagine a homogenous community that uniformly abides by its professed values. In addition, they actually or metaphorically distance themselves or rid "us" of unwanted or undesirable traits. All these "undesirable persons" are clustered together and seen as different and as a separate "them." This flawed interpretation by some members of faith communities—implying that HIV and AIDS are a punishment for sin—contributes to distancing people living with AIDS, changing these people from "us" to "them." This not only adds to the entrenchment of stigma and alienation of people living with AIDS but also makes the community sweep the issue under the carpet. The community's fixed notions of "us" and "them" erroneously identify AIDS as "their" problem, thereby denying the reality of AIDS. "How can I be one of 'them'? I am part of the 'Holy us'!" These lead to value-based assumptions made about morality and personal responsibility without accepting the reality that all people face vulnerabilities.

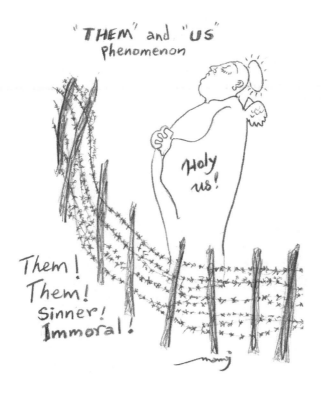

The historic "Global Consultation on Ecumenical Responses to the Challenges of HIV/AIDS in Africa," held in Nairobi, Kenya, in November 2001, expressed these concerns clearly in its "Plan of Action":

> We cannot speak of "them" and "us" when it comes to HIV/AIDS. The pain and fear of this disease have touched us all, but people living with HIV/AIDS are our greatest resource. We must no longer speak of "victims" in terms that diminish the courage, dignity and gifts of people living with HIV/AIDS. And we must be ready to work with all people of goodwill. We must now take up the responsibility to overcome stigma and discrimination within our own structures, while being a voice of moral strength demanding that our communities, nations and wider society respect the rights and dignity of people living with HIV/AIDS and condemn acts that stigmatise. The truth is that we are all made in the image of God. This means that discrimination is a sin, and stigmatising any person is contrary to the will of God.[4]

Love Your Neighbour as Yourself

The ethical mandate to "love your neighbour as yourself" (Lev. 19:18; Matt. 19:19; Mark 12:31) reflects the belief that all are created in God's image. Being the image of God is a relational issue. We are related and bound to God, but also to others. Jesus illustrates the "neighbour," in his parable of the good Samaritan (Luke 10:25-37), as one who is sensitive to the needs of the other and assists others in need. The neighbour could also be the one who is in need of assistance. Clarifying the question "Who is my neighbour?" means inquiring into one's identity in relation to the other and the quality of our relationship with each other. This quality of our relationship with others also defines our relationship with God. This relationship is tested in times of need. According to Matthew 25:31-46, Jesus expects us to see God and relate to God by responding to those who are vulnerable and on the margins of society: those who are hungry, thirsty, lonely, needing clothes, those who are incarcerated in prisons, or sick. We should note that Jesus *did not* describe the situation of those in need as famished, dehydrated, suicidal, stark naked, on death row, or terminally ill! He obliges us to be sensitive to the need of the "other," even before the situation gets really bad, and not to wait to respond until we are asked for help.

In the teachings of the Beatitudes (Matt. 5:1-11), Jesus encourages us to step outside our comfort zones. He calls us to be empathetic[5] to others and to respond with compassion, sincerity, and humility, promoting peace, showing mercy and courage, and striving for justice, even in the face of persecution.

One Body

This commitment also strengthens the vision of the whole community as part of one body of Christ (1 Cor. 12:12), however remote the part may be from us. We gather together as the body of Christ and work together in communion and in fellowship. The fellowship fosters in the community a connectedness that is characterized by compassionate and committed relationships. This interconnectedness implies that the welfare and well-being of the other are deeply significant to each one of us. There is no longer "us" and "them." If we are one body and we have one hand in fire and other in a bucket of water, can we claim that, on average, we are fine? We are called to accept that the virus affects us as a community. We are challenged to see that, as we all belong to the body of Christ, the suffering caused by HIV and AIDS affects all of us. We must recognize that the crisis of AIDS is our crisis and, as such, "Our church has AIDS."[6] The ecumenical movement has discussed profoundly the concept of "one body" in the context of HIV, as exemplified by the study process facilitated by the Cooperation of the Fellowship of Council of Churches in Southern Africa (FOCCISA) and Nordic Churches.[7]

HIV-positive church: The wounded bride of Christ

Professor Musa Dube, the pioneering and influential theologian who has effectively and consistently addressed HIV and AIDS in her writings and work (she was the first theological consultant to the WCC-EHAIA, from 2002 to 2004, and is a professor at the University of Botswana, teaching New Testament studies in the department of theology and religious studies), describes the HIV-positive church in a 2014 lecture:

> As an HIV- and AIDS-positive church, the African church chooses to identify with the "Other," who is vulnerable, who is marginalized, stigmatized, discriminated and oppressed. . . . The HIV-positive church is the wounded bride of Christ. She lives with the deadly virus upon her body and bears the marks of its opportunistic infections. She has experienced stigma and discrimination in her own home and among her family members. She is a church that knows suffering, death, grief. She is an orphaned and caregiving grandmother, and a midwife for a positive life. She embodies the least of these (Matt. 25:31-46).[8]

The body of Christ is HIV-positive

In the context of the unity of humanity, in the midst of suffering, being one body with Christ, when many of us are living with HIV, it has been boldly proposed that the "Body of Christ is HIV-positive."[9] The relevance of this powerful metaphor was addressed substantively and acknowledged by a global gathering of 140 church leaders, theologians, educators, and people living with HIV in 2011.[10] This concept is reminiscent of Jesus fulfilling the prophecy of Isaiah 53, becoming the man of sorrows, with the broken body and shedding blood for many. This is expressed powerfully in a thought-provoking painting, *Man of Sorrows: Christ with AIDS*, by the American artist and lay theologian Maxwell Lawton. The artist lived with HIV and died due to AIDS-related illness in 2006.

Who Can Separate Us from the Love of Christ?

In the statement of the WCC Central Committee titled "Churches' Compassionate Response to HIV and AIDS," in September 2006, the ecumenical leadership challenged churches and communities, quoting Romans 8:35: "Who can separate us from the love of Christ?" They asked the stark question, "Can HIV come between Christ and us? If someone attempts to come between HIV-positive

Man of Sorrows: Christ with AIDS—Maxwell Lawton (1956–2006)

In the Advent season of 1993, I was alone in my apartment and was overcome with grief from the loss of almost all my friends, loved ones and mentors to AIDS. I felt like no one knew me anymore. A strange thing happened as I cried; I had a waking dream, like a vision. I saw myself sitting on a hospital examination table, naked, and hooked up to oxygen and IV drips. Suddenly, the image changed. It was no longer me sitting there, but Christ, covered in AIDS cancer lesions with his head bowed, nude, wearing only a crown of thorns. I knew I had to paint it. I quickly gathered my supplies and, in a transcendent experience, I made the first version of *Man of Sorrows: Christ with AIDS*. I had questions that needed to be answered. As I painted Christ, I was reminded of the many versions of the "Man of Sorrows" referred to in Isaiah 53, 3-4, from the 16th century and of Gruenewald's Christ as a plague victim. This gave me the merit to continue. I also knew I had to answer the fundamentalists who were saying AIDS was God's judgment on gay people and drug users. In the painting, I also quoted Jesus' words from Matthew 25 that when you offer care giving "to the least of these, my brethren, you are doing it unto me." I intertwined the words with the image. Afterwards, I knew something inside me changed. I realized God knows my pain and shares my grief. I was healed of a lot of hurt. God still knew me . . .

In 1994, Archbishop Tutu and his new ministry, Wola Nani-Embrace, invited me to Cape Town to make a similar version of the painting in St. George's Cathedral. My painting brought attention to the AIDS crisis in South Africa. . . . I had many daily visitors while painting. Some were deeply touched. Others yelled and spit on me. When *Man of Sorrows: Christ with AIDS* appeared on the front page of the *Cape Times* in December 1994, it triggered worldwide controversy. When someone showed up at the cathedral "to rid the place of the heretic artist," I was placed in protective custody and Archbishop Tutu responded to the press, defending me and the painting as theologically correct.

The painting was seen by millions of people and was exhibited at the World Council of Churches and has appeared on numerous publications—Christian magazines, newspapers, periodicals, web sites, and books. The painting now hangs at Wola Nani-Embrace's center in Cape Town, where people still come to hear and see the message of hope and healing it offers.

—Maxwell Lawton, 2006[11]

people and God, does he or she come from God? Does the congregation make the person living with HIV feel welcome, loved and part of the same body? If the congregation perpetuates exclusion, avoidance, stigmatization or persecution is it not placing a barrier between God and God's children?"[12]

In the WCC study document *Facing AIDS: The Challenge, the Churches' Response*, the WCC consultative group on AIDS observed, "The very relevance of churches will be determined by their response. The crisis also challenges churches to re-examine the human conditions, which in fact promote the pandemic, and to sharpen their awareness of people's inhumanity to one another, of broken relationships and unjust structures, and their own complacency and complicity. HIV and AIDS are signs of the times, calling us to see and understand."[13]

Biblical teaching, the gospel of Christ, and the church traditions provide adequate frameworks for the church to train and to motivate its members to transform churches and communities to serve God's people in the midst of HIV and AIDS. It is clear that churches and communities need to pursue that route, to ensure that the negative interpretations of the religious texts, promoting fear, exclusion, and death are effectively countered.

Biblical Marching Orders

The biblical principles that have guided the ecumenical work in the field of HIV can be classified under five pillars:[14]

1. Don't judge

Jesus said, "Blessed are the merciful, for they will receive mercy" (Matt. 5:7), and in responding to the call to stoning the woman accused of adultery, he said, "Let anyone among you who is without sin be the first to throw a stone at her" (John 8:7). In the same vein, the apostle Paul wrote, ". . . you have no excuse, whoever you are, when you judge others; for in passing judgment on another you condemn yourself, because you, the judge, are doing the very same things" (Rom. 2:1). Many in the church have interpreted HIV and AIDS as God's punishment for sin, thus adding to the entrenched stigma and alienating people living with and affected by HIV and AIDS from receiving comprehensive HIV care. This approach is contradictory to Christ's teaching, as illustrated by his response to his disciples querying him as to whether a man was born blind as a result of his or his parents' sins: "Neither this man nor his parents sinned; he was born blind so that God's works might be revealed in him" (John 9:2-3).

The insistence on sexual purity as the exclusive solution to HIV and AIDS prevention while neglecting the biblical perspective of the sacredness of all human life has contributed to the tradition of silence and negative perception of human sexuality. This also has led to conflicting messages and unresolved approaches in the area of safer sex and HIV prevention.

The rich contribution of the ecumenical movement to the church's worship and liturgical life, and biblical reflection to help Christian congregations—such as the annual liturgies prepared for the World AIDS Day, anthologies of liturgies such as *Africa Praying*,[15] the 2007 Week of Prayer for Christian Unity focusing on HIV[16]—are great witnesses to the work under this pillar response to HIV.

2. Create safe spaces of grace: Transforming faith communities

Perhaps the most famous promise in the Judeo-Christian Bible is found in Psalm 23, where the psalmist expresses confidence in God's protection, saying, "Even though I walk through the darkest valley, I fear no evil; for you are with me," and concludes with "and I shall dwell in the house of God forever."

Faith communities and churches are mandated to be sacred sanctuaries of trust and confidentiality. They are to be:

- Spaces of grace that promote physical, psychological, and spiritual safety.
- Where one is without fear, shame, and intimidation.
- A place where one does not need to be guarded and intimidated.
- Where one can step outside one's own comfort zone.
- Where the integrity and dignity of each person are respected.
- A nonjudgmental space where one is accepted as one is.
- Where a person is seen beyond one's actions.
- Where one can be honest and the truth is spoken with love.
- A space for restoration and positive transformation.

HIV has highlighted the need for churches to be transformed into "safe spaces of grace," due to the root causes of HIV and the multiple factors that make individuals and communities vulnerable to HIV and its effects. The key issues that have benefitted from the ecumenical movement's attention include: human sexuality, gender relations and masculinity, and overcoming violence (especially sexual and gender-based violence). Perhaps the best example of a "safe space of grace" in action is the Contextual Bible Study movement, which gave birth to the Tamar Campaign.[17] The Contextual Bible Study (CBS) of Tamar's rape (2 Sam. 13:12-18) disrupts our collective silence on violence against women and brings about transformation and effective solutions. This study eventually developed into a campaign against gender and sexual violence. The Tamar Campaign helps churches to address sexual violence and violent models of masculinity. This grassroots initiative has been very effective in South Africa and has spread to other countries within Africa and to other continents. The WCC Ecumenical Theological Education programme has embraced the methodology since 2004. WCC-EHAIA has extensively used CBS to great impact and, because of the strong interconnectedness of sexual and gender-based violence (SGBV) with the HIV pandemic, since 2007 it has become widely popular. We will delve into the concept of "safe spaces of grace" in greater detail in chapter 4.

3. Serve those in need

According to Matthew 25:31-46, Jesus expects us to see God and relate to God by responding to those who are vulnerable and on the margins of society. Hence, service (*diakonia*) is seen as worship (*liturgia*). We are to discern the presence of God on the margins of society, amongst those who are vulnerable. We are to approach those in need with sincerity and deep respect and the willingness to learn from them, and also in partnership, to work together to find common solutions.

Jesus' overwhelming concern for the welfare of people is clearly indicated in his parting conversation with his disciple Peter (John 21), where he repeatedly asks Peter if he loves him. Each of the three times Jesus instructs Peter to "feed/ tend my lambs." Those who do not respond to the needs of the other are said not to conform with the love of God: "How does God's love abide in anyone who has the world's goods and sees a brother or sister in need and yet refuses help?" (1 John 3:17). Congregations and communities have a key role in accompanying people living with HIV. Currently, faith-based organizations (FBOs) are among the major health providers in developing countries, providing an average of about 40 percent of health services in sub-Saharan Africa. FBOs' core values lead them to offer compassionate care to people with a long-term commitment to societies, closely aligning with community needs.[18] The WCC has supported the development of Christian Health Organizations/Associations (CHAs) in more than 30 countries since 1968. The most substantial and successful of these structures work as national umbrella networks of church-based health providers. They coordinate and support the work of their members (including health providers and facilities and training institutes) through capacity building, advocating for a proper recognition of Christian health services, and negotiating with governments. Countries that have a CHA usually provide better data about the market share of Christian health work than countries without such an umbrella organization.[19] In 2007, with support from WCC, the African CHAs decided to form the Africa Christian Health Association Platform (ACHAP) as a coordinating hub. ACHAP represents the CHAs, fosters capacity building, joint learning, and exchange of knowledge among its members.[20] The ACHAP HIV/AIDS technical working group (TWG) is represented by HIV and AIDS programming experts from Kenya, Uganda, Tanzania, Zambia, Zimbabwe, Malawi, and Nigeria. The TWG serves as a technical reference group on HIV and AIDS programming related to prevention, screening, treatment, care, support services, and health systems necessary for effective HIV and AIDS programming. Partners working closely with the HIV and AIDS TWG include IMA World Health and the USAID-funded AIDSFree project, which, among other things, seeks to enhance pediatric care and treatment.[21]

The other key ecumenical organization is the Ecumenical Pharmaceutical Network (EPN), which was initiated in 1981 as the WCC's pharmaceutical programme to provide advice and consultation in the area of pharmaceutical services to church health programmes, particularly in Africa. Since 1997, it has become a global, church-related, independent organization, based in Nairobi. EPN seeks to strengthen the church pharmaceutical sector and enhance interventions that improve people's access to quality pharmaceutical services. They are actively engaged in advocacy, targeted at increasing access to and rational use of medicines.

In 2010 EPN published a very useful volume called *HIV and AIDS Treatment Literacy Guide for Church Leaders*. This book provides compelling insights into how church leaders can take up advocacy issues in matters of antiretroviral treatment as a life-prolonging intervention for people living with HIV, and deals with stigma and discrimination in the church.[22] EPN has also published and distributed HIV- and AIDS-treatment programme tools.

4. Speak truth to power

Give justice to the weak and the orphan;
maintain the rights of the lowly and the destitute.
Rescue the weak and the needy;
deliver them from the hand of the wicked. (Ps. 82:3, 4)

The prevalence, control, and impact of HIV and AIDS are usually much more than a matter of any individual contribution or one's lifestyle or behavioural patterns. Significant societal and structural reasons behind the vulnerabilities are driven or made worse by imbalanced gender relations, violence, poverty, and the lack of access to comprehensive HIV care, including diagnostics and treatment.

The lack of access could be because of financial disparities, macroeconomic conditions set by unfair trade practices and agreements, or because of stigma and discrimination at the societal and health-facility level. The advocacy by faith communities for reducing the cost of treatment for HIV and the campaigns for greater access to pediatric antiretroviral preparations, as well as the advocacy of ecumenical and denominational initiatives against violations of the human rights of key affected populations, are good examples of the actions taken under this principle.

5. Build strong foundations of faith

Like the wise man who built his house on the rock in Jesus' parable of the wise and foolish men (Matt. 7:21-27), the ecumenical movement aspires to build church ministries on solid foundations. Narrowmindedness, insufficient knowledge and skills, denominational divisions, and lack of networking amongst denominations, with governments, and with other NGOs have been a major impediment to the churches in their response to HIV and AIDS.

Initially, the ecumenical movement focused on spreading necessary and current information on AIDS for pastors and congregations. Then the discussion progressed to consultations on pastoral care and pastoral counselling and the development and sharing of resources material to equip congregations for compassionate and competent response to HIV. In the focussed efforts to bring transformation to the budding pastors and theologians, the ecumenical movement invested in developing HIV-sensitive theological curricula in different regions. It also facilitated the publication of critical collections of theological reflection addressing the root causes of the pandemic such as stigma and discrimination; sexual and gender-based violence; transformative masculinities and femininities; and sexual reproductive health and rights, among others.

Called to Heal and to Be Healed

Churches are called to heal and to be healed in the context of HIV and AIDS. Being called to be healed means that churches must reflect, repent, and rededicate themselves to the gospel of Christ. In order to abide by Jesus' commission to preach, to teach, and to heal, God calls the churches to be healing communities in a world that is characterized by brokenness through war, injustice, poverty, marginalization, and disease. The biblical teaching, the gospel of Christ, and church traditions provide adequate frameworks for the church to train and to motivate its adherents to serve God's people in the midst of HIV and AIDS.

The teachings of Jesus, especially in relating with the other, are unequivocal and clear. We are to love our neighbours as ourselves, and to see the divine in the other, especially those on the margins of society. We are to respond to the needs of society and those in need with empathy, compassion, and a sense of urgency. We are to desist from being judgmental, to address the contexts that make people vulnerable, and to look at the responsibility of society, beyond personal responsibility. It is our responsibility to ensure that we work to make our faith communities and congregations and families into spaces of grace, make available educational approaches and creative tools for all ages that are inclusive and welcoming so we can address issues that make people vulnerable to HIV, and contribute to positive transformation in the lives of individuals and society.

Chapter 3

Living with HIV

All nations of the world have committed themselves to end the AIDS epidemic by 2030 as part of the Sustainable Development Goals set forth by the United Nations. Ending the AIDS epidemic will require extraordinary efforts in leadership, investment, and focus, both over the short term and the longer term, to deliver even more services and even greater social change. In anticipation of this challenge, UNAIDS launched a global Fast-Track Initiative, on World AIDS Day 2014. But societies will be able to achieve these targets only if people who live with HIV are not stigmatized and discriminated against. HIV-related stigma and discrimination refers to prejudice, negative attitudes, and abuse directed at people living with HIV and AIDS. In 35 percent of countries with available data, over 50 percent of men and women report having discriminatory attitudes toward people living with HIV.[1]

The consequences of stigma and discrimination are wide ranging. Some people are shunned by family, peers, and the wider community, while others face poor treatment in healthcare and educational settings, erosion of their human rights, and psychological damage.[2] These all limit access to HIV testing, treatment, and other HIV services.[3] The People Living with HIV Stigma Index[4] indicates that roughly one in every eight people living with HIV is being denied health services because of stigma and discrimination.[5]

Ultimately, the effectiveness of a HIV programme in a community and a country is largely decided on how the society treats people living with HIV. So the life experiences of these people are central to our quest to understand the ecumenical journey with HIV and AIDS.

Millions of Children of God

People living with HIV have always been on the frontline of the struggle to overcome HIV. Much has changed from the early days of the epidemic in the 1980s, when no treatment was available, and when the world was paralyzed with fear and ignorance. Today, we have made considerable progress. The availability of comprehensive HIV care, which includes good preventive methods, effective and simple testing, and effective treatment has converted HIV from a "death sentence" to a preventable chronic disease. Of the nearly 37 million people living with HIV as of June 2015, 15.8 million are accessing HIV treatment. Although an estimated 30 million new HIV infections have been averted in the past 15 years due to the scaling-up of services, there were 2 million new HIV infections and 1.2 million AIDS-related deaths in 2014. Of all the people estimated to be living with HIV, nearly half do not even know their HIV status!

These figures reveal the many challenges that people living with HIV continue to face. The high levels of stigma, discrimination, and ignorance discourage people from testing for HIV and seeking comprehensive care. The total numbers can also be misleading, as the burden of disease is highly variable between different age groups and diverse communities. For instance, at the epicentre of the HIV epidemic in southern Africa, adolescent girls and young women aged 15 to 24 contribute a disproportionate 30 percent of all new infections and seroconvert five to seven years earlier than their male peers.[6] Exploitation by older men, susceptibility to violence and coercion, paucity of education, and economic insecurity and dependence all contribute to this vulnerability.

"Same-sex-loving people,"[7] along with other vulnerable communities, face a devastating HIV epidemic globally. Prevalence among same-sex-loving people has been found to be as high as 25 percent in Ghana; 30 percent in Jamaica; 43 percent in coastal Kenya; and 25 percent in Thailand.[8] It is estimated that by 2020, 42 percent of all new HIV infections in Asia will occur among same-sex-loving people.[9] The high levels of discrimination and the violation of the rights and dignity of girls, young women, and persons belonging to vulnerable communities contribute to poor access to comprehensive HIV services.

Confronting God in the Midst of Suffering

In the struggle to overcome HIV and for the message to get across, it is vital that HIV be seen as a condition faced by real people with lives and dreams, and not just a challenge clothed in overwhelming statistics and smart strategies.

The progress in the journey that the world has made with regard to HIV has been at a heavy cost of human lives. Millions have carried the cross of AIDS. From the era before treatment was accessible, we uphold the precious memory of those who were lost to the pandemic. The AIDS Memorial Quilt is a powerful visual reminder, consisting of more than 48,000 individual memorial panels commemorating the lives of persons who have died of AIDS, having been sewn together by friends, lovers, and family members.[10] Additionally, these images have been digitized and made available on the AIDS Memorial Quilt web site, enhancing display activity and HIV-prevention education programmes.

The other significant experience in remembrance has been "memory work." This is an innovative and effective approach to psychosocial support and accompaniment of children, women, and men affected by or infected with HIV and AIDS. The term *memory work* refers to a number of group-oriented therapeutic methods that enable people to examine their life stories and to cope with disease, death, and grief.[11] The experience of the Sinomlando Centre for Oral History and Memory Work in Africa, a Pietermaritzburg-based organization involved in memory work for orphans and vulnerable children since 2000, is one significant example.[12]

There have been many pioneers who lived with HIV and who are no longer with us. Ernesto Cardoso (1957–1995) was an inspiring Brazilian Methodist lay theologian, musician, and composer who profoundly influenced the worship life of the church worldwide. He composed famous songs such as "Momento Novo" ("New Moment"), "Canto do Povo Reunido" ("Song of Reunited People"), "No Amor de Deus" ("The Love of God"), and many others that speak of the liberating grace of God and the communion which is built in the encounter with those labelled as "others."

Cardoso coordinated the Latin American Council of Churches (CLAI) Liturgy Network and worked with the Institute for Religious Studies (ISER). He was diagnosed as HIV-positive in 1990. As a member of the World Council of Churches' Consultative Group on HIV, he had a crucial and inspirational role in the development of ecumenical policy on HIV. He died of AIDS-related illness in 1995 at the age of 38. Just before his death, he reflected on the life of the prophet Job. His reflections are published in the WCC study document *Facing AIDS: The Challenge, the Response*:

> I remember the absurd amount of suffering Job went through and how, at the end of his experience, doing theology with his own body, he learned to reject rationalizations imposed as truths. I also remember that his misguided friends expected Job to trust them, accept the pain, confess his sin and, hopefully,

be forgiven and cured! At the end of Job's experience, seeing the Sacred in all grandeur, Job exclaims: "Hear, and I will speak; I will question you, and you declare to me. I had heard of you by the hearing of the ear, but now my eye sees you" (Job 42:4, 5).

Hope and resurrection are intimately related to his profound experience of faith. The impact of this confrontation usually cannot be expressed in words; a radical change of perception is required. In this dramatic situation, many people are seeking a home, a shoulder, an embrace, and meaning that helps them to understand this pain, to face it, and go beyond resignation. They wish to integrate it as a part of life's experience, daring to advance and extend the limits imposed by illness.

The attitude of the leadership of the churches, its thinkers (theologians), and its ministers (deacons and pastors) should help, and not undermine, people. They should assist the multitude of homeless, lonely, tired, and desperate people to recover and to reencounter God from the context of their suffering. Only confronting the divine mystery and being open to the revelation of God can help. Well-prepared speeches are no longer convincing; let us learn to worship. Symbols, gestures, and silence are fundamental: learning to do liturgy with people who suffer, learning to discover signs of the sacred in the midst of rejection. We must learn to recognize this "holy land," to remove one's sandals, and, in silence and profound expectations, to meet like Moses what is "further beyond"![13]

Ernesto Cardoso yearned for a transformed world, where we discover new, fresh ways of relating, shaking off old habits and hypocrisy. These thoughts, as reflected in his prayer titled "Prepare our hands for a touch," have left an indelible impact on ecumenical consciousness.

God of Life,
prepare our hands for a touch,
a new and different touch.

Prepare our hands for a touch,
a touch of encounter,
a touch of awakening,
a touch of hope,
a touch of feeling.

Many are the worn-out gestures.
Many are the movements frozen in time.
Many are the useless excuses just to repeat attitudes.

Give us daring
to create a new community,
new kinds of affection,
breaking away from old ways of relating,
encouraging true, meaningful ways to move into closeness.[14]

The lives of the innumerable martyrs have inspired many into action. These include many of the young lives lost in the early days of the epidemic, which had a profound effect on many and precipitated policy change. Nkosi Johnson (1989–2001), a South African child living with HIV and AIDS, had a powerful impact on public perceptions of the pandemic and its effects before his death at the age of 12. He was born HIV-positive, and was adopted by a woman named Gail Johnson, because his biological mother, debilitated by the disease, was unable to care for him. Nkosi's birth mother died of AIDS in the same year that he started school. His condition steadily worsened over the years, although, with the help of medication and treatment, he was able to lead a relatively active life at school and home.

Nkosi was the keynote speaker at the 13th International AIDS Conference, where he encouraged people with HIV and AIDS to be open about the disease and to seek equal treatment. Nkosi finished his speech with these words: "Care for us and accept us—we are all human beings. We are normal. We have hands. We have feet. We can walk, we can talk, we have needs just like everyone else—don't be afraid of us—we are all the same!" Nelson Mandela referred to Nkosi as an "icon of the struggle for life."[15]

As the narrative of "A Prophet called Doubt" below will reveal, my own journey with HIV was indelibly influenced by a dying child.

A Prophet Called Doubt

In January 1999, I joined the World Council of Churches as the staffperson responsible for the "Health and Healing" programme. The challenge of responding to the call of churches in sub- Saharan Africa, given to WCC at its eighth General Assembly in Harare (1998), to accompany them in facing and overcoming the HIV and AIDS pandemic weighed heavily on me. As a Malaysian medical doctor trained in public health, I had extensive community-based experience in health in different regions in India and in working with faith communities. Yet, it was my first opportunity to face the full force of the AIDS epidemic. In that year an estimated 34.3 million people were living with HIV; approximately

2.8 million people died of AIDS and AIDS-related illness. Half a million of those who died were children. Care and support packages were only accessible according to resource availability in each context and only a negligible number of those needing treatment received antiretroviral treatment.

The magnitude of the suffering I witnessed, my sense of inadequacy, and lack of resources and experience made me feel helpless, paralyzed, and depressed. The fact that I was the lone health-related staff member replacing a bigger team of experienced individuals made the challenge even more onerous.

But in the very first year at the WCC, with the understanding and solidarity of colleagues such as Rev. Jacques Matthey and Rev. Dr Nyambura Njoroge, I was able to work with and come in close contact with individuals, churches, and communities in Africa. This relationship transformed me by enlightening me with a greater vision for humanity. Without romanticizing suffering, the resilience, love, hope, and courage of individuals, churches, and communities in Africa spurred me to break free from my numbed resignation.

I consider one particular experience during that period a turning point in my journey with HIV. In 1999, I was in Zimbabwe to assist and co-organize the Pan African Conference of Christian Health Associations. After facilitating this conference, I found time to visit some programmes that churches were implementing as responses to the HIV and AIDS pandemic. As part of those visits, I visited the Emerald Hill Children's Home in Harare, run by the Dominican Missionary Sisters of the Sacred Heart of Jesus, which housed around 100 children, most of them orphans. Many of these children were orphaned as a result of the AIDS pandemic and some of them were also living with HIV. On the day of my visit, the mood in the children's home was heavy with sadness. One of the children at the home, a much-loved 11-year-old boy, was dying due to AIDS-related complications and no access to antiretroviral therapy. The boy's name was "Doubt." I had heard of many children named after positive virtues: Hope, Joy, Grace, Mercy; I even knew of a Happy. But this was the first time I encountered a child called Doubt. The sad religious sisters told me that Doubt was an exceptional child. He was very loving and helpful, always thinking about the welfare of others before himself.

I asked if I could see him. Since I was trained as a physician, seeing a dying child was not an unfamiliar experience for me. But the encounter with Doubt made an indelible impression on me. He was lying on a clean bed in a well-kept, bright room. Sister Tarisai was sitting by his side, caring for him. He was thin and gaunt. Though he was 11 years old, he was not bigger than a 7-year-old child. His eyes were striking. Unlike most people who are dying, his eyes, though set in sunken orbits, were bright and sharp. We looked at each other for a long time, and held each other's hands, but did not speak.

After I left, Doubt remained vividly in my mind. I reflected on my encounter and visualized him in the context of the vision of the prophet Ezekiel in the Holy Bible, where Ezekiel prophesized and brought to life, through the power of God, dry human bones heaped in a valley, converting them to a vigorous and live army of people (Ezek. 37:1-14). Doubt was the prophet. I was among the heaps of dry bones in the valley. He addressed me:

I am an orphan;
I have HIV and AIDS;
I am dying;
But I have HOPE, I have COURAGE.

You are not an orphan;
You do not have HIV and AIDS;
But you are not just dying;
You are already dead!
For you have no HOPE nor COURAGE!

My trip to Zimbabwe was a turning point. The prophet called Doubt helped me to see with clarity. He made me realize that the bottom line is not my capacity or incapacity; rather, it is the need of the community that has to be met. He helped me to recognize and acknowledge people who are on the margins of society. I realized that those who are vulnerable and facing tremendous challenges are precious resource persons and teachers, and not just recipients of services. This encounter taught me to ask for help and to work with those who are attempting the same. Together, we made networks of trust to bring about a positive change in people's lives through compassionate and competent action. Together, I realized we could respond to existential challenges better, faster, and more inclusively. With both African and global leaders, I could play a part in mobilizing churches in Africa, Asia, and other regions of the world to intensify the efforts in overcoming HIV and AIDS in a comprehensive manner.

Doubt died two days after my visit, but the prophet called Doubt lives on in my heart to this day.

—Manoj Kurian

Silent No More

Coming face to face with tremendous suffering does not always initiate or strengthen people's faith in God. Elie Wiesel, writer, political activist, Holocaust survivor, and Nobel Peace Prize laureate, was once a budding Talmud scholar in the rural Hungarian village of Sighet. But as a 15-year-old boy, in the spring of 1944, his small community was torn asunder and the residents transported to the Nazi concentration camp at Auschwitz. He lost his mother, his beloved little sister, and his father in the Holocaust. In his first book, *Night*, published in 1958, while narrating that harrowing experience he questions the existence of God. No one who has read *Night* can ever forget Wiesel's description of the scene where the Gestapo hanged a small child, who was too light to die from hanging.

> But the third rope was still moving: the child, too light, was still breathing.
> . . . And so he remained for more than half an hour, lingering between life and death, writhing before our eyes. And we were forced to look at him at close range. He was still alive when I passed him. His tongue was still red, his eyes not yet extinguished. Behind me, I heard [a] man asking: "For God's sake, where is God?" And from within me, I heard a voice answer: "Where is He? This is where—hanging here from this gallows . . ."[16]

Twenty-eight years after writing this book, in his Nobel Peace Prize acceptance speech in Oslo, Eli Wiesel began with words of gratitude to the Creator, reciting the prayer: "Blessed be Thou . . . for giving us life, for sustaining us, and for enabling us to reach this day." After surviving the Holocaust, he swore never to be silent whenever and wherever human beings endure suffering and humiliation. He memorably added, "When human lives are endangered, when human dignity is in jeopardy, national borders and sensitivities become irrelevant. Wherever men and women are persecuted because of their race, religion, or political views, that place must—at that moment—become the centre of the universe."[17] In our context, to the list of reasons for persecution that we need to battle, we would add disease, HIV status, sexual orientation, and gender.

I believe that Elie Wiesel, like Job, played a prophetic role by questioning God. His disturbing question raises the important role of individuals and society in creating life-giving and life-destroying circumstances. The burden of upholding hope and faith in difficult times should never rest solely with the persons experiencing vulnerability and suffering. It is the corporate responsibility of the wider society to provide an enabling, inclusive, and loving environment.

Father Robert Igo, OSB, in his thought-provoking article "Making Sense of Suffering," states, "Suffering may want to declare that God does not exist, but the very absence of God does not provide an answer either. Only love provides a convincing reply to the question why."[18] Are the churches and congregations replying to the question with love?

Positive Lives

When the environment empowers a person living with HIV to live openly and when brave women and men who are living with HIV take up the challenge, many possibilities and avenues to overcome the pandemic become available. Key issues can no longer be dismissed as if they do not concern the community. People living with HIV give society the possibility of relating to the reality of HIV and related issues in a more forthright manner. Their presence and leadership enable church groups and communities to discuss HIV and AIDS, health, sexual behaviour, and issues related to religion and culture more freely and openly.

Their lives also demonstrate that being HIV-positive is not a cause for shame or despair, or reason to buckle to discrimination. The presence of high-profile religious leaders among those who are HIV-positive can also help reduce HIV-related stigma within faith communities, by demonstrating that they can also live positively and openly with the virus, serving God even more meaningfully and effectively than before.[19]

Living openly as HIV-positive also gives them the possibility of connecting with and developing peer groups and "positive networks." These positive groups provide mutual support and mentor those who are positive, but facing difficulties. The resulting solidarity and support also helps to combat the crippling self-stigma, which reinforces societal stigma.

The Gideon Effect

Evidence suggests that, just as with the celebrities Rock Hudson and Magic Johnson disclosing their HIV-positive status, the Hollywood actor Charlie Sheen's recent disclosure (17 November 2015) may similarly be reinvigorating awareness and prevention of HIV. Scientists have called this the "Charlie Sheen effect,"[20] and are keen to leverage this increased interest in HIV to promote discussion and awareness regarding HIV. The disclosure by high-profile individuals linked to faith and churches that they are living with HIV has had a profound and sustained positive impact in the struggle to overcome HIV.

The positive global influence of the prominent and inspiring figure such as Rev. Canon Gideon Byamugisha, can be considered as the "Gideon Effect." A priest in the Church of Uganda, he became the first religious leader to declare that he is living with HIV after he was diagnosed HIV-positive in January 1992, at the age of 32 years, following the death of his first wife. After intense discussions with close family members, he decided to disclose his HIV-positive status publicly.

Canon Gideon's sincere, compassionate, confident, and forthright witness has had a huge impact in the struggle against HIV in the faith context. A brilliant orator and a warm and approachable person, he never fails to inspire and enthuse his audiences. He has authored numerous articles and books about HIV and Christian theology.

In the early years of the pandemic, people living with HIV (and their leaders who were HIV-positive, too) were much less visible. "Everywhere I was going, people were saying, 'Meet Canon Gideon, the first religious leader to open up about his HIV status.' And I asked myself, 'Where is the second leader to open up? Where is the third?'" Increasingly, people living with HIV started seeking Canon Gideon's support and guidance, especially from the year 1998 onwards. The obvious need for solidarity for (and with) religious leaders living with HIV led him and other pioneers such as the Rev. Fr. J. P. Mokgethi-Heath, Rev. Christo Greyling, and Rev. Phumzile Mabizela (among others) to co-found the African Network of Religious Leaders Living With and/or Personally Affected by HIV and AIDS (ANERELA+), launched officially in Kampala, in October 2003. The movement has since spread to other regions and in 2006 evolved into INERELA+ (International Network of Religious Leaders—lay and ordained, women and men—Living with or Personally Affected by HIV). INERELA+ has 16 active country networks in the African region and also has a presence in Asia/Pacific, Canada, the Americas, Europe, and Central Asia.

Canon Gideon was instrumental in devising two now-famous acronyms that sum up his practical and essential strategies for achieving an AIDS-free world. The first of these, SAVE, stands for Safer practices, Appropriate treatment and nutrition, Voluntary Counselling and Testing, and Empowerment. But standing in the way of these strategies is a barrier of formidable obstacles, which he summarizes as SSDDIM: Stigma, Shame, Denial, Discrimination, Inaction, and Mis-action. The SAVE prevention methodology has been used and taught by INERELA+ for over eight years and is available as a comprehensive toolkit. The toolkit provides users with a step-by-step methodology for addressing sensitive issues in an open, informative, and nonstigmatizing way that does not avoid otherwise difficult issues.[21]

Canon Gideon Byamugisha's message has achieved even a wider audience through a film the Strategies for Hope Trust and Christian AID produced in

2004, entitled *What Can I Do?* This film tells the story of how he first learned of his HIV-positive status, how he came to grips with it, and then developed a ministry that has given hope and inspiration to millions of people.

Canon Gideon Byamugisha's achievements have received national and international recognition, for instance, through the Parliament of Uganda Award (2008), the Niwano Peace Prize (2009), an honorary doctorate in divinity from the University of Botswana (2010), the Archbishop of Canterbury's Cross of St Augustine (2012), and the appointment as a visiting professor of political science at the University of the South, Sewanee, USA (2013).

At every opportunity, Canon Gideon Byamugisha makes it a point to remind people of the individuals, groups, and organizations that have stood by him, empowering him to live openly and positively with HIV. There are many lives that have made the "Gideon effect" a reality, illustrating the importance of a supportive community for a person living with HIV to live a successful and fulfilling life.

- His sister-in-law Eunice, who was the wife of the principal of the theological college where he studied and was teaching at the time of his diagnosis, for disclosing the fact that his wife had passed way due to an AIDS-related illness and encouraging him and standing by him after he was tested positive for HIV.

- His students at the theological college for accepting him as a teacher and mentor.

- Bishop Samuel Balagadde Sekadde, of the Diocese of Namirembe, who after being told of Gideon's HIV status, in 1995, welcomed him and made Gideon the head of the Diocese's HIV programmes and interventions. In 2001, Bishop Samuel proposed Gideon's name to the diocesan council among the six reverends he was proposing to elevate to the honorary title of "Canon of St Paul's Cathedral, Namirembe," for Gideon's exemplary leadership and unique defense of faith in the time of HIV. The diocesan council members who received the proposal and other Christians who heard about it welcomed it with ululations and with the famous hymn of praise among Eastern Africa Christians: "*Tukutendereza Yesu*" ("We Praise You Jesus!")

- His family—which includes his brothers (led by Mr Paddy Nahabwe), his sisters (led by Mrs Winnie Abaho), his mother, Christine, his wife, Pamela (who is HIV-positive) and three daughters, Patience (born to his late first wife), Love, and Gift (whom he had with Pamela). The couple decided to have Love and Gift after drugs to prevent transmission of the virus from mother to child became available in 2000. All his children are free of HIV.

- His friends, various supporters, and well-wishers among ecumenical bodies, faith communities, networks of people living with HIV, and among development partners (who individually and collectively channel moral, financial, and technical support to him through the Friends of Canon Gideon Foundation—FOCAGIFO)

Be Right and Safe!—Rev. Canon Gideon Byamugisha (2009)

We are confusing the word "right" with the word "safe." Most Christian ethics is not about what is "safe" and "unsafe." Most of it is about what is "right" and "wrong." The mentality and moral reasoning of the Christian world has been found wanting when it comes to HIV and AIDS. It is not ready to deal accurately with AIDS because it brings moral attributes of what is "wrong" and what is "right" in sex and sexuality and transplants them on to AIDS.

They are imposed on the HIV and AIDS prevention conversation and people conclude that when you do the morally "right" things in sex then you are safe from HIV, without considering other variables like unsafe environments. Not all "sexual saints" are free from HIV and not all "sexual sinners" are HIV-positive! There should be an ethic that tells people to do what is "right" and "safe" in both sexual and nonsexual matters at the individual, family, local community, national, regional, and global levels. But even now there is a false way of thinking that suggests that what is "right" in moral categories is automatically "safe" in sexual, reproductive, and public health terms, and that what is "wrong" in Christian morals is automatically or inherently "unsafe."

So, when people say, "You are HIV-positive?" then their next question is, "Oh, what wrong thing did you do? Did you commit adultery? Were you unfaithful, promiscuous, or a prostitute?" It is like saying, "You have typhoid—whose water did you steal?" or "You have mosquito bites all over your body and affected by malaria parasites—whose bed did you sleep in without their permission?" or "You had a car accident—whose car did you steal?"

Indeed, not all sexual sinners are HIV-positive and not all sexual saints are HIV negative. People who feel they are good, right, and faithful will not think about AIDS risk and vulnerability as their problem. They will have a false security in a world where millions of "good," "well-behaved," and "faithful" people are already HIV-positive and yet their HIV status does not automatically show either on their faces or in the good, right, and faithful things they do! And there is nothing worse than that: to think you are secure when you are not.[22]

How Did You Get It?—Rev. Fr. J. P. Mokgethi-Heath, Policy Advisor on HIV and Theology, Church of Sweden

The question always asked has been "How did you get it?" and the only reason people ask this question is simply to determine "Are you innocent or are you guilty—do we have to find a way of accommodating you or can we simply write you off as someone who is deserving of judgement?"

The reality is that this moral stance to HIV is what erodes the self-worth of people. Within the faith community we preach about, we teach about human dignity! We celebrate the way in which we can say we are all created in the image and likeness of God, and yet so much of what we do erodes self-worth.

It was while attending the 10th International Congress on AIDS in Asia and the Pacific (ICAAP) meeting in Busan that I for the first time heard of the research which had been done on the "Syndemic Construct." A group of you MSM [men who have sex with men] were questioned, and there were six questions they needed to answer:

1. Have you been rejected by your family because of your sexual orientation?
2. Have you experienced rejection from your faith community on the grounds of your sexual orientation?
3. Have you ever abused substances?
4. Have you tried to commit suicide?
5. Have you sold sex?
6. Have you experienced physical, sexual, or emotional abuse?

Now if we look at these questions, they are all areas that we as faith community can engage in to reassure people, to restore the self-worth of the individual. THIS IS OUR CORE BUSINESS, and yet, more frequently than not, we are part of the problem rather than being part of the solution. And it is this negative self-image which manifests itself as vulnerability to HIV. And if we are the source of that vulnerability, then we must also accept culpability.

HIV is a virus, not a moral condition! I first said this in 2006 during the UNGASS in New York. It was during the early days in trying to get the role and place of the faith community's engagement with HIV more recognized. And in many senses we are still not there. I like to tell people that this is a lesson we can learn from HIV: HIV simply does not discriminate. HIV does not ask, Do you live in Africa or Europe? It does not ask, Are you heterosexual or homosexual? HIV is not interested in whether you are male or female, rich or poor, young or old, what country you come from, which language you speak, or any one of the myriad attributes we as humans use to differentiate between people. All HIV asks is: IS THERE AN ENTRY POINT. That's it. Nothing more. Our moral judgments will not save people; rather, they will continue to create vulnerabilities simply because we emphasize the wrong things. What we need to do is build communities of inclusion, and eliminate vulnerabilities to HIV. That we can do, it costs nothing, and yet it is the most costly intervention. It means accepting change, challenging our "comfortability."

When we first developed the SAVE methodology in INERELA+ our main focus was on trying to get people to understand that HIV is not all about sex. We believed that if we could disassociate HIV and sex we could, to a large extent, challenge the stigma around HIV. I still believe this to be true, but acknowledging that the vast majority of HIV transmissions are sexual means also having to confront sexuality. This remains a thorny issue for faith communities. But unless we can come to a place where we do not tolerate but rather celebrate this wonderful God-given gift, we will never have the tools to empower people to make good and informed decisions for themselves about their own sexual health, not least of which is the steps they need to take to protect themselves and their loved ones from HIV.[23]

Life-Giving or Life-Destroying Circumstances?

Gracia Violeta Ross Quiroga, co-founder and leader of Bolivia's first national network of people living with HIV and AIDS, is a global leader representing women living with HIV. Before testing HIV-positive in the year 2000, as a rebellious, young university student she had lived a lifestyle that made her vulnerable and suffered sexual abuse.

As the daughter of an evangelical pastor in Bolivia, disclosing her HIV status presented the risk of facing blame, guilt, and condemnation. But she found acceptance and love in her family. Her family received her with open arms; they told me they did not want to know what happened, they just wanted to be with her and support her until the last day.

Touched and pacified, she was reminded of the promise from Psalm 103:13: "As a father has compassion for his children, so the LORD has compassion for those who fear him." She still experiences this love as a reflection of God's love in her own family. "In my anguish due to the HIV-positive diagnosis, I looked for God again. God gave me freedom from blame and shame, I found peace, forgiveness, hope, and eternal life. The Lord consoled me in the worst time of my life, giving me the strength to go on. God showed me nothing could take me away from the divine and incomparable love, neither the evil I had committed, the evil that was perpetuated on me, nor the virus, nor even death."[24]

But, unfortunately, in Bolivia and many countries around the world, Gracia Violeta's experience is the exception rather than the rule. People living with HIV still face oppressive levels of stigma and discrimination, at all levels of society. The intensity of the stigma increases greatly when the person is a same-sex-loving person, and if the person is transgender or involved in sex work. Though nearly 16,000 people are living with HIV, the National Network of Bolivian People Living with HIV and AIDS has only 200 members, and only 15 persons are open about their status. This, despite the fact that all people living with HIV in Bolivia are eligible to receive free treatment. Gracia speaks with anguish: "Most people living with HIV in churches do not feel secure to disclose their HIV status. Most congregations still do not know the basics about HIV and there is still a lot of fear and intolerance. There is universal treatment, but people living with HIV are sad, fearful, and lonely. Very few people have a home. We still have a long way to go and there is no room for complacency!"[25]

Life Is Important: My Life Is Valuable When I Am Still Alive—Pornsawan Christpirak (Thailand)

My marriage life was very short. We separated after being together for three years. I knew that I was infected with HIV in 1998 when I was very sick and got admitted to a hospital due to many complications in my health condition. I was affected by cytomegalovirus (CMV) in my eyes that causes blindness. My body weight went down from 47 kg to 29 kg only. I got pneumonia and started coughing blood. My tongue was cracked and painful. I could not eat nor breathe and needed a respirator.

I got HIV from my husband because he used injecting drugs. When I knew I got HIV, the first feelings were of shock, fear, regret, disappointment, and not knowing, not understanding why it had to happen to me because I had not been involved in any inappropriate or risky behaviour. I have been a devout Christian since I was a child. I went to church and studied the Bible to serve God. I chose my husband from a Christian College who had a similar belief in the religion. Why did this have to happen to me? I was sorrowful and cried in the hospital. I didn't want to meet or speak to anybody.

Impact on family members

I had believed that no matter what serious disease I have, my people will never leave me because they are my beloved people. God taught me to face the difficult situation. I believe God allowed me to lose all my help and shelter so that I would focus on the Almighty, who is loving and caring and who has the power to give or take life.

My family did love and cared for me. But my mother, brothers, and sisters have a hard life, and they were limited in their ability to assist me. When I was admitted to the hospital for an extended period, my mother had to struggle hard to come every day to look after me. Later, she had to stop coming. I experienced very lonely moments. I yearned for my family members. I missed them so much. I wanted to hug my children but couldn't. I had to send my children to a Christ Foundation for around three years.

Sufferings of living with AIDS

I felt most stressed when I had to be away from my two beloved sons, as I had to undergo treatment to cure my complicated diseases. Stigmatization and judgmental attitudes from other people branded me as a promiscuous woman who got HIV because I lived an immoral life. It was unbearable that even Christians stigmatized, accused, and blamed me. I had to be in the spotlight where many people looked at me with disgust as if I wasn't a human being at all. No one dared to hug me. No one dared to eat with me. There were only gossip and bad rumours. I couldn't look in a mirror because I couldn't bear to see the change. My face and skin had changed. No one could recognize me. I became another person. I was stressed with many complications of the disease that I had, not knowing when I would recover, where I would find money to buy medicine, and how I could live without being a burden to my family.

My hope and encouragement to fight against AIDS

My first encouragement in this world are my two sons. I didn't want to die then because I still wanted to live and raise them to be good people. I didn't want them to be orphans. The additional encouragement was from my family. But, it's Jesus Christ who is my greatest friend and my best physician who performed a miracle by curing me through doctors in the hospital and medicines.

The things that I wanted to do when I get stronger

I promised God that if I recovered and would be better, I would go back to finish studying the Bible and serve Him all my life. I would take my children from the Foundation to take care of them myself and teach them to be good people.

The most important were to help friends, who are living with HIV and AIDS with no other support, and to encourage them to have faith and begin a new life.

Lessons learned from my life

My life is valuable while I am still alive, and of double value when it is lived for family members and friends. All obstacles, problems, and sicknesses that happen to us are temporary. They come one day and go away on another day. They don't stay forever. Everything has its period. Don't worry. Be mindful and handle it cautiously.

Even though HIV will always stay in our blood because there is no medicine to treat it permanently, don't be afraid because we know we can handle it. If we are careful and disciplined in taking medicines, it cannot attack us. We should be concerned about our health and have regular check-ups so that when there is a disease, we will know about it in the early stages and can treat it in time.

Life is meaningful. Do good things when we are still alive because when we are sick, even if we want to do something, it's not easy to do so.

Being infected with HIV doesn't lower the value of humanity. We still have rights and can do many things. When I recovered from my sickness, I went back to study until I got two Master's degrees. Everybody told me that I got AIDS and would die soon, but I wasn't discouraged. I am now a pastor in Adonai Church.

Glory Hut Foundation

Some people I know took me to the Glory Hut Foundation. When I first entered the foundation, I felt warm, like I'm not abandoned. Now I am responsible for the foundation and we have three shelters in Pattaya, Thailand, to take care of sisters and brothers who are living with HIV. They live in harmony, supporting each other, and have become a big family in Jesus Christ. Praise the Lord![26]

Nothing about Us without Us: Partnership and Leadership

The ecumenical movement strives to ensure the greater and meaningful participation of people living with HIV in all HIV-related discussions and policy development and programme implementation, as elucidated in the UNAIDS Denver Principles of 1983.

The WCC developed a key document, "Towards a Policy on HIV/AIDS in the Workplace: A Working Document," in 2005, to assist member churches and ecumenical organizations to update their polices to ensure that people living with HIV are protected in the institutional workplaces associated with churches and related organizations. This was developed per international norms and standards set by the International Labour Organization. Many churches and global ecumenical networks, such as the World Alliance of YMCAs, used these principles to update the workplace policies of their member institutions and national bodies.

The need and importance of people living with HIV to develop their own organizations, caucuses, and networks—both in the secular and the religious contexts—were recognized by the ecumenical movement. The WCC, in order to assist the fledgling African Network of Religious Leaders Living with and/or Personally Affected by HIV and AIDS (ANERELA+), hosted their staff in the various regional offices of WCC-EHAIA during the early days of the movement. In collaboration with the Global Network of People Living with HIV (GNP+) and ANERELA+, WCC also developed critical background information and guidelines for member churches and ecumenical organizations to equip them for developing partnerships with networks of people living with HIV. Andrew Doupe, representing the GNP+, played a critical role in developing and promoting these transformative policy documents.

It was also clear that, just as in the secular world, the rights and dignity of people living with HIV are to be guarded diligently. HIV-related stigma is seen to be at the heart of many failed efforts over the years—both church and secular—to respond to HIV, particularly to break the silence and denial surrounding the existence of HIV in communities. Many interventions, whether for HIV prevention, care, support, or treatment, have also been less than effective due to HIV-related stigma. The WCC specifically worked to assist churches in a transformation process (that in some cases had already begun and in others was yet to begin), and to steer that process. They are targeted at all levels of the church, whether church leaders, parish priest or ministers, people working in faith-based organizations, and so forth. The policies developed helped churches deal with the issues that confront churches and organizations for people living with HIV in their attempts to forge partnerships, to assist in helping make partnerships functional and effective. The documentation also lifted up some of the good practices and partnerships and also highlighted dangers, when relationships could go wrong. Concrete information on an array of issues which need to be addressed, such as confidentiality, tokenism, capacity building, and monitoring and evaluation, were also provided.

The Denver Principles[27]

The Denver Principles laid out in 1983 by people living with HIV are a witness to their struggle for self-empowerment. The principles are still relevant and powerful today as they were then. They asked people to be called "People with HIV and AIDS," rather than victims.

The Denver Principles recommend that everyone protect people living with HIV from stigma, discrimination, and from being blamed for the epidemic or being generalized about their lifestyles. They also recommend that people living with HIV and AIDS

- Form caucuses to choose their own representatives, to deal with the media, to choose their own agenda, and to plan their own strategies.

- Be involved at every level of decision making and specifically serve on the boards of directors of provider organizations and to be included in all AIDS forums with equal credibility as other participants, to share their own experiences and knowledge.

- Substitute low-risk sexual behaviors for those that could endanger themselves or their partners and show an ethical responsibility to inform their potential sexual partners of their health status.

They also demanded the rights of people living with HIV and AIDS
1. To live as full and satisfying sexual and emotional lives as anyone else.

2. To receive quality medical treatment and quality social-service provision without discrimination of any form, including sexual orientation, gender, diagnosis, economic status, or race.

3. To receive full explanations of all medical procedures and risks, to choose or refuse their treatment modalities, to refuse to participate in research without jeopardizing their treatment, and to make informed decisions about their lives.

4. To privacy, to confidentiality of medical records, to human respect, and to choose who their significant others are.

5. To LIVE—in dignity.

Framework for Dialogue

In the spirit of making the faith communities accountable to the people living with HIV, theological networks, and the international community, a "Framework for Dialogue" emerged from the Summit of High-Level Religious Leaders held in the Netherlands in March 2010. The Framework for Dialogue is a tool for developing joint actions and ongoing discussions between religious leaders, faith-based organizations, and networks of people living with HIV at the national level.

The idea was to replicate the successful format of a dialogue between religious leaders and people living with HIV on a national level. Four international partners—Ecumenical Advocacy Alliance (EAA), Global Network of People Living with HIV (GNP+), International Network of Religious Leaders Living with or Personally Affected by HIV and AIDS (INERELA+) and UNAIDS—came together in early 2011 to move the concept of the Framework for Dialogue from an idea to a reality. This process has now been successfully implemented in numerous countries in Africa and in Asia.[28]

You Will Know Societies by Their Fruits

The greatest achievement of any society would be to ensure that the least privileged and those who are vulnerable in the community experience equity, justice, and accompaniment. In the context of HIV, the quality of life experienced by those living with HIV and those vulnerable to acquiring HIV is indicative of the maturity, competence, and compassion of the society. Faith communities have lots to contribute in achieving this ideal.

> [Jesus said,] "You will know them by their fruits. Do men gather grapes from thornbushes or figs from thistles? Even so, every good tree bears good fruit, but a bad tree bears bad fruit. A good tree cannot bear bad fruit, nor can a bad tree bear good fruit. Every tree that does not bear good fruit is cut down and thrown into the fire. Therefore by their fruits you will know them." (Matt. 7:16-20)

It is vital that communities be intentional in ensuring that people living with HIV are well taken care of and that they do not experience stigma, discrimination, or violation of their human dignity and rights.

Chapter 4

Safe Spaces of Grace

The world has made much progress in conquering HIV. We know much more about the virus itself. We have made headway in developing many drugs that work against the virus. We know how to prevent and treat the disease effectively. Although a cure is yet to be discovered, HIV has been converted into a chronic disease. We look forward to the day when HIV is no longer a threat. But it is important to note that the factors which make us vulnerable to HIV will most likely remain as they are if we do not address them in a forthright manner. Even if we eradicate HIV, its place will be taken up by yet another malady should we continue to be silent on aspects of our life and society that make us vulnerable to HIV. But do our communities provide the safe space for people to address this vulnerability? This chapter delves into the nature and practice of "safe spaces for grace" as vital venues to address the various domains of our life that make us vulnerable.

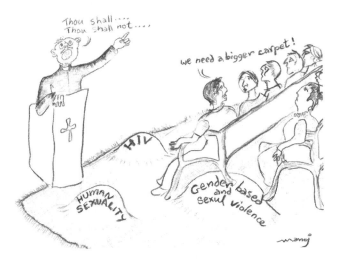

HIV in the Context of Vulnerability

The ecumenical movement has helped churches and communities to understand HIV and AIDS in a holistic manner. It is clear that HIV and AIDS are an expression of a fragmented world and a broken society. The disease is but a symptom of a wider malady, a curtain that, when drawn back, exposes society's weaknesses and challenges. But HIV and AIDS have also given us an opportunity to address many issues that we have generally avoided, to our long-term detriment. It is important to identify the various forms of vulnerability that have put us at risk for acquiring HIV and AIDS. Individual and community experiences of vulnerability include situations of powerlessness. Vulnerability indicates a situation in which something or someone can be hurt or wounded; exposed to danger or attack; or is unprotected. To be vulnerable in the context of HIV and AIDS implies that one has limited or no control over one's risk of acquiring HIV or, for those already infected with or affected by HIV, have little or no access to appropriate care and support. Vulnerability is the net result of the interplay of many factors, both personal (including biological) and societal.[1] In theological understanding, it is Jesus Christ who exemplarily shows us at the cross the utmost vulnerability we face in our faith: the moment of feeling abandoned even by God (Matt. 27:46).[2] Yet God does not let God's servants down. In the suffering, death, and resurrection of Jesus, we find our mission for Christian HIV and AIDS work. The ecumenical movement has helped communities to examine the domains that need to be addressed to reduce the vulnerability of people to HIV and AIDS in the context of our faith. The key domains include:

1. Gender relations and masculinity
2. Human sexuality
3. Violence (especially sexual and gender-based, including abuse within intimate relationships)

But these issues are seldom discussed openly. The topics can be very divisive for faith communities, so it is vital that there be openness and a nonprescriptive approach, both of which promote open discussions to prepare the ground for positive transformation. The ecumenical movement has strived to secure safe spaces of grace in faith communities to address critical issues. To deal with these issues with any degree of helpfulness, churches and communities need safe, trustworthy, and nonjudgmental spaces. These safe spaces also need to be consistent, inclusive, and dependable spaces in which to discuss and act on the key issues.

Features of Safe Spaces of Grace

We have already had an initial discussion on the topic of "safe spaces of grace" in chapter 2, but now I will go into some additional detail. The features of safe spaces of grace[3] can be described as follows:

- The presence of knowledge and skills on HIV and AIDS and related issues.

- Opportunities for critical dialogue and debate about HIV and AIDS and related issues.
  - Possibility to renegotiate understanding and theology, with the flexibility to interrogate dogma and moral norms with a view toward encouraging social action to deal with the issues.
  - Possibility to renegotiate behaviour and identities, facilitated in a non-judgmental environment where there is a building up of self-esteem and self-worth.

- A sense of individual and collective ownership of the problem and responsibility for contributing to its solution.

- Confidence in the existence of individual, group, and community strengths which could be mobilized to fight the epidemic.

- A sense of solidarity among group members around tackling HIV and AIDS and related issues. This solidarity is qualified with some key qualities such as:
  - space is trustworthy and one that keeps confidentiality;
  members feel they are listened to, accompanied, supported, and mentored; does not make one more vulnerable.

- Strong links with potential support agencies in the public and private sectors outside of the community (bridging or linking social capital).

- Inclusivity and the ability to bridge across power gradients.
  - Creating the space for all to participate and contribute irrespective of all potential markers of difference.
  - To link and connect between groups within the faith community with the possibility of influencing transformation regarding the issue at hand across the community.
  - To be aware of power dynamics and differentials that could smother the safe space. For example, between women and men, minority and majority, resident and migrant, and so forth.

- Recognize that the source of grace is God.

The safe space of grace is where one receives the other unconditionally, in the presence of God, with all their differences, deficiencies, and strengths as a fellow sojourner in this life. We acknowledge that all fall short of the perfection of God, and we do not merit God's grace. Hence, each of us, as a child of God, is loved by God and sit around the same table, relating with each other with humility and respect, recognizing our mutual vulnerabilities and flaws. "But God proves his love for us in that while we still were sinners Christ died for us" (Rom. 5:8).

In various Christian traditions, "grace" can be described as the love and mercy that is given to us by God because God desires us to have it, not because of anything we have done to earn it. In the Orthodox Christian tradition, grace is also identified with the uncreated energies of God. These point to the great potential for positive societal transformation, provided we are open to and do not reject the grace of God. The safe spaces of grace require the creation of a space for reflection, for listening, for relational conversations, providing space for God's grace to bring about transformation. This also provides the milieu for serving, empowering, and loving others; building relationships of trust; and facilitating change from within. This space recognizes God's love for the creation and God's will to reconcile and heal the broken relationships with the world. This perspective begins with the understanding that it is God, not human beings, who has taken the initiative to show God's love to the creation. We respectfully provide the space.[4]

Five Levels on Which Safe Spaces of Grace Function

I would describe safe spaces of grace as manifested and experienced on five levels.

1. *Governance and leadership space* is where awareness and experience on the issues will enhance the possibility that decision makers and those in the various hierarchies will introduce policies that are conducive to the promotion of safe and dynamic spaces in faith communities, thus promoting healthy, informed, and balanced societies. Many of the successful series of consultations that took place over the last three decades, bringing forth key statements, declarations, policies, and plans of actions, as described in chapter 1, depended on this space.

2. *Ethical and theological space* is where the analysis, teachings, practice, dogma, celebrations, spirituality, worship, and liturgies provide the

possibility for the issues concerned to be addressed in a helpful manner. Theological institutions also provide this vital space for theological analysis, and publications compile key thinking that promotes this process. The WCC's Ecumenical HIV and AIDS Initiative in Africa (WCC-EHAIA) has played a leading role in the transformation of theological thinking on HIV. With Prof. Musa W. Dube as its first theology consultant, followed later by Prof. Ezra Chitando and Rev. Charles Kaagba, WCC-EHAIA began facilitating the mainstreaming of HIV in theological programmes. Musa Dube's *HIV/AIDS and the Curriculum: Methods of Integrating HIV/AIDS in Theological Programmes* (2003)[5] and Ezra Chitando's *Mainstreaming HIV and AIDS in Theological Education: Experiences and Explorations* (2008)[6] have been used widely in theological institutions and university departments of theology, religious studies, and other faculties of theology. These key materials equipped the ethical and theological space and facilitated graduates of African theological institutions to become effective agents of change in the time of HIV.

Contextual Bible Studies (CBS) are a vital methodology that can be used at all the four levels, but that work to bring about the possibility of renegotiating understanding and theology, with the aim of bringing about social action to deal with the issues of concern.

3. *Community safe spaces* are where systems, principles, and practices are in place to promote discussion of the issues involved and actions are taken to address challenges. These are where critical, perhaps even hurtful, concerns can be freely discussed and considered, without fear of repercussions. A community safe space is where people are able to fully express themselves, without fear of being made to feel uncomfortable, unwelcome, or unsafe on account of sex, race/ethnicity, sexual orientation, gender identity or expression, cultural background, religious affiliation, age, or physical or mental ability. They are places where the rules guard each person's self-respect and dignity and strongly encourage everyone to respect others. These spaces could be quasi-governmental or actual governmental bodies, educational institutions, and civil-society spaces.

4. *Congregational safe spaces* are where traditional and innovative systems, principles, and practice are in place to promote discussion of the issues involved and actions are taken to address challenges. These could be youth, women's, and men's groups, Sunday schools, religious schools, or

seminaries. These could also be denominational, interdenominational, or interreligious spaces.

5. *Family safe spaces* are where equity, safety, and the sacredness of relationships are promoted and sustained and abuse is prevented.

Equipping Churches and Communities to Develop Safe Spaces of Grace

The WCC-EHAIA has been equipping churches and congregations to become compassionate and competent churches, through their extensive workshops and a wide spectrum of resource material. They provide information on mainstreaming HIV into the life of the church and on building HIV competence through such volumes as Sue Parry's *Beacons of Hope: HIV Competent Churches—A Framework for Action* (2008) and *Practicing Hope: A Handbook for Building HIV and AIDS Competence in the Churches* (2013). Other resource materials, such as Musa W. Dube's *A Handbook on HIV/AIDS Sensitive Sermon Guidelines and Liturgy* (2003); Robert Igo's *Pastoral Counselling: A Christian Response to People Living with HIV/AIDS* (2005) and *A Window into Hope: An Invitation to Faith in the Context of HIV and AIDS* (2009); and Ezra Chitando's *Living with Hope: African Churches and HIV/AIDS* (2007) and *Acting in Hope: African Churches and HIV/AIDS* (2007), are designed for reflection and transformation throughout the churches, from the leadership to the congregation level.

The Key Domains

Gender relations and masculinity

Young girls

Young girls are much more vulnerable to HIV. In southern Africa, which is the region of the world that is most seriously affected by HIV, adolescent girls and young women aged 15 to 24 contribute a disproportionate 30 percent of all new infections and seroconvert five to seven years earlier than their male peers.[7,8] Exploitation by older men, susceptibility to violence and coercion, paucity of education, economic insecurity and dependence all contribute to this vulnerability. Abduction and forced marriages are also common in many countries, and completely violate a woman's choice not only in choosing her sexual partner, but also her decision to be sexually active or not.[9] Various church-led initiatives, educational institutions, and activities led by church-related organizations such as the YWCA focus on providing the space, educational opportunities, and training to empower young women and girls in reducing their vulnerability. Comprehensive sexual education and quality sexual and reproductive health services are essential parts of securing this space. The World YWCA's work on ending child marriages is also a significant movement to protect girls form deprivation, disease, disability, and death.[10]

A significant experience of a safe space of grace is the Circle of Concerned African Women Theologians (hereafter the Circle). The Circle was established in 1989 in Accra, Ghana. In the year before that, Mercy Amba Oduyoye, the noted Ghanaian ecumenical leader and past Deputy General Secretary of the WCC, organized a group of female African theologians to form a planning committee. The key objectives of the Circle are research, writing, and publishing on women's issues in the realm of religion and culture. The Circle has registered over 800 members on the continent and abroad. The criterion for membership is the commitment to research, write, and publish on issues affecting African women and women of African descent in religion and culture. The Circle is the space for women from Africa to do communal theology based on their religious, cultural, and social experiences. It draws its membership from women of diverse backgrounds, nationalities, cultures, and religions rooted in African Indigenous Religions, Christianity, Islam, and Judaism. It encompasses indigenous African women and seeks to relate to African women of American, Asiatic, and European origins. These concerned women are engaged in theological dialogue with cultures, religions, sacred writings, and oral stories that shape the African context and define the women of this continent. The vision of the Circle is to empower African women to contribute their critical thinking and analysis to advance current knowledge. Theology, religion, and culture are the three chosen foci, which must be used as the framework for Circle research and publications.

Since 2003, WCC-EHAIA has developed a close partnership with the Circle's history of researching HIV, gender, and religion. The most significant research output from the partnership of the Circle and WCC-EHAIA is *Compassionate Circles: African Women Theologians Facing HIV*,[11] which indicates where the gaps are in the Circle research and writing in the area of gender, faith, and HIV and AIDS in Africa. Through this effort, future Circle researchers were challenged to broaden their research, including a shift in focus from women to also include men.[12]

Widowhood

Evidence suggests that, in many regions, compared to never-married women, widowed and married women are significantly more likely to be HIV-positive.[13] Society expects women living with HIV who are widows to be celibate, but expectations of widowers living with HIV may not be that restrictive[14] and, hence, there are more challenges regarding remarriage. Certain deleterious cultural practices in many regions such as widow inheritance and cleansing make widows highly vulnerable to HIV.[15] While church-run programmes are very much accessible to women, especially in the rural areas, the patriarchal attitudes undermining women in many Christian communities render them more vulnerable.

Have You Heard Me Today?[16]

Woman 1: I am Eve, the bone of your bone, and the flesh of your flesh.
Woman 2: I am Sarah, the woman who calls you Lord and master.
Woman 3: I am Hagar your maidservant; your unofficial wife, expelled from your house.
Woman 4: I am Leah, the woman you married against your will.
Woman 5: I am Dinah, your only daughter, who was raped by Shechem.
Woman 6: I am Tamar, your desperate widow who plays the sex worker.
Woman 7: I am Ruth, your young widow sleeping at your feet, asking for your cover.
Woman 8: I am Bathsheba, raped by your king and married by the same.
Woman 9: I am Vashti, your wife banished so that all women can obey husbands.
Woman 10: I am the Levite's concubine, raped by the mob and cut up by my lover.

ALL Women:
We are the broken women of the Hebrew Bible.
We are broken women in a broken world.
We are women searching for our own healing.
Have you heard us today?

Woman 11: I am Mary, the pregnant woman with no place to go.
Woman 12: I am the Samaritan woman, with five husbands and none for her own.
Woman 13: I am Martha, the woman who is cooking while you sit and talk.

Woman 14: I am Mary, the woman who silently anoints your feet with oil.

Woman 15: I am the street woman, washing your feet with my tears.

Woman 16: I am the bent-over woman, waiting for your healing touch.

Woman 17: I am the bleeding woman, struggling to touch your garment of power.

Woman 18: I am Anna, the widow praying for liberation in your temple.

Woman 19: I am the persistent widow in your courts, crying, "Grant me justice."

Woman 20: I am Jezebel, the demonized woman, blamed for all evil.

ALL Women:

We are women of the Christian Testament.

We are broken women in a broken world.

We are women searching for our own healing.

Have you heard us today?

Woman 21: I am the woman in your home, I am your wife.

Woman 22: I am the woman in your house, I am your lover, your live-in girlfriend.

Woman 23: I am the woman in your life, I am your mother.

Woman 24: I am a woman in your workplace, I am your secretary.

Woman 25: I am a woman in your streets, I am your sex worker.

Woman 26: I am a working woman in your house with no property of my own.

Woman 27: I am the woman in your life with no control over my body.

Woman 28: I am the woman in your bed with a blue eye and broken ribs.

Woman 29: I am the woman raped in your house, streets, offices and church.

Woman 30: I am the woman in your church, cooking, cleaning, clapping and dancing.

ALL WOMEN:

We are women of the world.

We are Women of Faith.

And we are secular women.

We are women seeking for our own healing.

Have you heard us today?

Masculinity

The notion of "crises of masculinity" refers to multiple processes of social, economic, and cultural change that undermine and challenge traditional men's roles and forms of masculinity. Men are often victims of the expectations that society places on them. The patriarchal norms of the church add to their challenges. The HIV epidemic has posed serious threats to men and masculinity. Sexual-behaviour studies globally indicate that men—whether married or single, heterosexual, homosexual, or bisexual—have higher reported rates of partner change than women. Also, men are more likely to have multiple partners simultaneously, more likely to have a sexual partner outside of their regular or long-term relationship, and more likely to buy sex. In many cultures, variety in sexual partners is seen as essential to the nature of men. In practice, this means that men will likely have more sex partners on average than women. Conversely, women are expected to be sexually passive, and are discouraged from acquiring knowledge about sex, suggesting condoms or other contraceptive use to men, or accessing sexual and reproductive health services. Many of the world's women have little power to negotiate safer sex, including when, with whom, and how sex occurs.[17] Because the HIV epidemic is a gendered phenomenon, as is now generally acknowledged, then the response to the epidemic should also be gender-based and thus involve men and address questions of masculinity. The challenge has been about how to continue to challenge and provoke for more responsible masculinities, without slipping into stereotyping and generalizing masculinities and problematizing male sexuality as the source of high-risk behaviour and sexual aggression.[18] WCC-EHAIA has brought to its focus "Transformative Masculinities and Femininities" by developing theological resources and scholarship and incorporating the topics into its training programmes.

Transgender people

The needs of transgender people within the global HIV epidemic remain largely unmet, although steps are being made to redress this. Issues such as social marginalization, violence, lack of access to basic services, and substance use contribute to significantly higher rates of HIV and STIs; the current situation in India has been presented to underscore this. In Peru, a recent study about access to services for people living with HIV found that the majority of transgender people surveyed have relatively low levels of education and employment, lack health insurance, and often do not have access to personal documentation. Strategies for best practice among trans populations include grounding the work in the community, acknowledging the role of race and ethnicity, being culturally appropriate, increasing access to healthcare, as well as developing and supporting staff.

In a qualitative report by RedLactrans and the International AIDS Alliance, on the situation of transgender women in 17 countries in Latin America, the main findings are:

- The systematic nature and scope of the human-rights violations committed against transgender human-rights defenders and other transgender women by state actors.

- Deeply rooted transphobia, namely fear or hatred of transgender people, across state structures at every level.

- This facilitates a similarly systematic climate of impunity with regard to human-rights violations committed against transgender activists and other transgender women.

- According to Colombian activists, 60 transgender women were murdered between 2005 and 2012 without a single person having been brought to justice.[19]

Recent systematic review and meta-analysis that assessed HIV infection burdens in transgender women in 15 countries (USA, 6 Asia-Pacific, 5 Latin America, 3 Europe)[20] shows that the odds for transgender women to get infected by HIV across all 15 countries was nearly 50 times more than that of all adults of reproductive age.

The churches largely do not provide any space for these marginalized communities. In 2004, at a church leaders conference convened by the WCC and the Church of South India, Noori, a transgender woman leader living with HIV, challenged the attendees, quoting from Isaiah 56:4-5, saying that God loves her more than all the leaders present. She appealed to Christian congregations to help all transgender persons to get employed and to help to advocate for their acceptance so that they are not forced into sex work as their only available means of livelihood.

For thus says the LORD:
"To the eunuchs who keep my sabbaths,
who choose the things that please me
and hold fast my covenant,
I will give, in my house and within my walls,
a monument and a name

better than sons and daughters;
I will give them an everlasting name
that shall not be cut off." (Isa. 56:4, 5)

Human sexuality

Human sexuality is how people experience and express themselves as sexual beings. Biologically, sexuality can encompass sexual intercourse and sexual contact in all its forms, as well as the physiological and psychological aspects of sexual behaviour. Sociologically, it can cover the cultural, political, and legal aspects; and philosophically, it can span the moral, ethical, theological, spiritual, or religious aspects.

So, sexuality is much more than sexual feelings or sexual intercourse. It is an important part of who every person is. It includes all the feelings, thoughts, and behaviours of being female or male, being attracted and attractive to others, and being in love, as well as being in relationships that include sexual intimacy and physical sexual activity.

Sexual ethics in the Judeo-Christian tradition and teachings

The guidelines for sexual ethics from the Judeo-Christian tradition and teachings are twofold. One part, the "property ethic," is where one's spouse is categorized along with other property; the sin of violation is greed, leading one to trespass against the property of one's neighbour (see the Ten Commandments in Exod. 20:2-17 and Deut, 5:6-21). The second part is a "purity ethic." Purity means avoidance of dirt or that which is not proper or that which is disorderly. This avoidance has had a deep influence on popular morality across cultures. The elaborate rules that evolved are given in the books of Deuteronomy and Leviticus. These give the boundaries of human behaviour, be it dietary, marital, or sexual, so as to ensure purity of the individual and the community, as a people who are set apart by God.[21]

The Jesus revolution and Christian back-tracking

Jesus Christ's teaching was revolutionary, as the community he strived for was not limited by purity codes. The teachings reject the age-old link between physical purity and access to the relationship with God. This does not mean that the concepts of purity and impurity were abolished. The demand for purity was elevated beyond superficiality and actions to one's very thought processes and intentions. Jesus also turned topsy-turvy the hierarchies of relationships and of power. By making the child the model for entry into the reign of God, as opposed to the father, Jesus attempted to negate the structures of society and the hierarchies that govern them.[22] The gospel promotes equality between men and women as they stand before God's grace. This was practically applied as the early Christian movement was marked by the active and independent involvement of women who were either married or single. Jesus also reiterated marriage as a union of flesh, normally irrevocable except by death. The wife was no longer disposable (divorceable) property. Instead, husband and wife were understood as human equals, who now constitute one flesh. This principle also brought sexual union into the family in a new way that rivaled existing family structures that revolved around the "property ethic" of the patriarch. In this new paradigm, sexual life and property are always subordinate to the reign of God.

But through the centuries, many old "purity and property ethics" have been reinforced and new boundaries have been created, which goes against the spirit of Jesus' revolutionary teachings. A notable contribution to the puritan ideology of repressed sexuality dates back to the fifth-century church father and theologian Saint Augustine, whose concept of "original sin" became dogma: sexual desire is sinful; infants are infected from the moment of conception with the disease of original sin; and Adam and Eve's sin corrupted the whole of nature itself.

The political and cultural goals of the theocratic movements have been to delegitimize and censor all forms of human sexuality that do not fit into the accepted mold: "sex between a man and woman who are married, in the strict patriarchal format that was approved by the church." Other expressions of sexuality are sinful and must be repressed or even punished. To that end, the theocratic movements seek to see sexuality exclusively as a means for procreation, criminalize homosexuality, promote abstinence-only sex education, and advocate censorship.

So sexuality has been subjected to the power equations that have been used to control and predict societal behaviour, and the community has been one of the key channels of this control. But in the light of the taboo nature of discussions of sexuality within many church settings, those who self-identify as "holy" people are prevented from developing new and creative ways of talking about sex and HIV transmission.[23]

Holistic Praxis

The ecumenical space has the potential for each narrative of each child of God to be valued deeply and acknowledged respectfully. The diversity of opinions and realities of the fellowship and the provision of safe spaces for dialogue and respectful listening give rise to fresh ideas and perspectives. This contributes to the responsive development of creative initiatives at different levels that have a positive impact on people's lives. Unfortunately, this unity has not been fully and meaningfully realized and experienced in a number of areas, human sexuality being one of the most significant. In fact, even the foundation of the unity of many churches has been threatened.

Human sexuality incorporates many issues, such as sexual orientation, gender identity, sexual relationships, and reproductive and sexual health. The greatest threats to the principle of "one people" have been the issues of sexual orientation and of women's sexual and reproductive health, which often narrowly boil down to ethical issues about abortion. This is because, while the known majority of people are heterosexual, inappropriate and often repressive and intolerant responses toward nonheterosexual persons consume too much of the limited space that is available for discussions on human sexuality in ecumenical faith communities. The extreme reactions associated with the response to homosexual relationships often act as a smoke screen to cover up and avoid addressing the many issues with which the community needs to deal—sexual violence and abuse, incest, or rape and violence within the supposedly sacred spaces of family, marriage, and church. Notwithstanding the existing gender disparities, women are ethically still viewed as perpetual minors who have no real capacity to go through moral-discernment processes without the control and intervention of the churches.

But communities of faith, listening and learning from each other, comforting, coping, and overcoming crisis are not divided among those of different sexual orientations. Recognizing that lesbian, gay, bisexual, transsexual, and intersexed (LGBTI) individuals are a living part of the community of faith is critical. The fact that we are all children of God, reflecting our Creator and worthy to be accorded the same worth, respect, and dignity, compels us to strive against all violations of human rights, including those perpetrated against sexual minorities. The "campaign of love" (as captured in the letter of the WCC general secretary to Ugandan president Yoweri Kaguta Museveni raising concerns regarding the Anti-homosexuality Bill, 2009)[24] that the WCC has engaged to challenge homophobia and unjust laws targeting homosexuals is a good example of the result of such a conviction and is in keeping with the principle of "one people" that defines the ecumenical movement. "One people" does not mean heterosexual people but, rather, an inclusive community that respects sexual diversity. People of different sexual orientations are part of the living community, contributing to the richness and diversity of society.

But discrimination and criminalizing homosexual orientation and consensual relationships infringes on the ability of individuals and groups to live dignified, safe, creative, and fulfilling lives. Whoever stands in the way of the love of God and people does this against the will of God (Rom. 8:35). Keeping silent in the face of injustice and cruelty and compartmentalizing our spirituality and praxis is not an option for people of faith within the ecumenical movement.[25] There are many examples of WCC member churches and national and regional councils of churches that provide the inclusive, safe spaces of grace for holistic discussions on human sexuality.[26]

Rev. Godson Lawson, a pastor in the Methodist Church in Togo and the chair of the international reference group of WCC-EHAIA, guides the work especially in the West Africa region. Reverend Lawson, along with the WCC-EHAIA regional consultant, Ms. Ayoko Bahun-Wilson, accompanies communities who have a high prevalence of HIV and are very vulnerable to HIV, such as same-sex-loving people, transgender communities, and people who inject drugs. They are working hard to engage the churches fully in this work and to develop chaplaincies for the churches' work outside congregations in different areas of need. They have also created observatories, with the full involvement of People Living with HIV, to monitor stigma and discrimination.[27]

HIV-Positive, Gay, and Gospel Artist George Barasa

George Barasa is Kenya's first and only gospel musician who is open both about his HIV status and his sexual identity. From his teenage years, Barasa developed a career as a gospel singer and photo model. In 2011, when he was only 19 years old, his sexuality became a public issue when *The Star* newspaper revealed his sexuality. Subsequently, he was disowned by his family and had to quit school, after which he moved to Nairobi and, through many struggles, managed to build his career, under the artist name Joji Baro. He decided to use his public outing by *The Star* as a platform to care no longer about the opinions of others but to be open about his sexuality and HIV status: "I decided to come out about my status and my sexuality to save myself from the agony and pain of living a lie. . . . I just want to leave this world a better place than how I found it whereby someone won't have to introduce themselves as 'Hi Am Gay and am HIV+.'"[28]

In recent years he has deliberately broadened the scope of his work and he calls himself an "artivist"—the word he uses to describe his work as an artist engaged in activism. Most of his activism focuses on sexual health and LGBTQI rights in Kenya and in wider Africa. Among other things, he was invited to contribute to conversations with faith leaders on human sexuality, hosted by the WCC-EHAIA in 2015. Most recently, in February 2016, he released a video clip that he directed, telling the story of his life and making a political statement about the experiences of gay and lesbian people in Africa. Entitled *Same Love*, the clip ends with a paraphrase of 1 Corinthians 13:4-5, stating:

Love is patient,
Love is kind,
Love is selfless,
Love is faith,
Love is full of hope,
Love is full of trust,
Love is not proud,
Love is God and God is love.

Through his experiences, Barasa has been able to rediscover the meaning of his Christian faith as essentially being about love. That belief is the inspiration for his artistic and activism work as Kenya's first and only openly gay, HIV-positive gospel singer who wants to make a difference in the world.
—Adriaan S. van Klinken

Violence, especially sexual and gender-based, including abuse within intimate relationships

A dialogue between then-Archbishop Rowan Williams and Michel Sidibé of UNAIDS

Michel Sidibé: "It is unacceptable that one in three women around the world will be raped, beaten, coerced into sex, or otherwise abused in her lifetime.

"We must recognize again this year that women and girls still face the higher risk of infection—and why, gender inequity is the fuel that feeds the fire of violence against women and girls, and it is both a cause and consequence of women's increased vulnerability to HIV.

"In many societies, women and girls face unequal opportunities, discrimination, and human rights violations. And while laws may exist on the books to protect their rights and give them greater opportunities, these rights aren't always fulfilled or supported by society and its leaders—including faith leaders."

Referring to a specific message from Gracia Violeta, a survivor of rape, he said, "I agree with Violeta that it takes more than prayer to heal and empower women who have endured sexual violence—to transform them from victims to survivors. It takes compassionate leadership that reaches beyond scripture and traditional rites and teachings." *He added,* "While the church—or the synagogue, temple or mosque—can be a rock-solid source of unmoving strength to a community, it must also be able to respond sensitively to the needs of women who have been hurt. For example, can an institution whose leaders are almost always men truly perceive the fears and hear the voices of women at risk of violence? And when it advocates for strong families, can it appreciate that the danger to women and girls often lurks inside their own homes? Do care, support and justice extend to women who sell sex or use drugs? Or who are transgendered? Yes. There should be no line that distinguishes who deserves and who does not. Women who have been victims of violence need many things: To have their dignity restored and to be protected from stigma and shame. To ensure their attackers brought to justice. To have access to psychological and medical care, including sexual and reproductive health. And ultimately, to be empowered, like Violeta, as leaders in achieving full equity in their worlds. My question to Archbishop Williams is this: beyond prayers and spiritual comfort, what more can the church offer to survivors of sexual violence?"

Dr Rowan Williams, Archbishop of Canterbury: "Gracia Violeta's letter is moving and disturbing. You are quite right to underline the concerns it raises about how religion can sometimes reinforce violent and oppressive attitudes to women, how it can help to silence honesty and protest, and so can make even worse the position of women who are at risk of and from HIV infection.

"What can be done? A lot has already been initiated to challenge the distorted theology that can underlie violent or collusive behaviour. Many churches I know have taken the biblical story of the rape of King David's daughter Tamar as a starting point for rethinking their approach and clarifying the unacceptability of the male behaviour depicted in this and other stories. If we are to make progress here, we have to expose toxic and destructive patterns of masculinity. And for cultures steeped in the Bible, it is important to start by showing that the Bible does not endorse or absolve violence against women.

"But in addition, there needs to be a coherent and persistent message about breaking the silence. The 'Silent No More' campaign has found wide support; and the launch in 2011 of the 'We Will Speak Out' coalition[29] of faith groups and faith leaders, in the wake of the research done by Tearfund's Silent No More, has proved a benchmark for challenging communities and leaders who fail to see this as a priority. Our own Anglican archbishops from DR Congo, Rwanda and Burundi have had a leading role in this. And last year's conference of Anglican primates issued a full and robust statement on gender-related violence which has now been strongly reaffirmed by the global Anglican Consultative Council. These policy statements rest on a lot of impressive grassroots practice, linking survivors to medical, legal and counselling support, and local livelihood training schemes—and also naming and shaming the culture of impunity, especially the impunity of those who in any way exercise power, in churches or elsewhere. But so often in my own travels I have found the most important service the Church can offer is to be a place where it is safe to speak about what has happened. Last year in DR Congo, and more recently in a Church-based centre in Papua New Guinea, I had the painful privilege of spending time with women who had accessed the services offered by the Church and were finding a new voice and new courage to confront those who had humiliated and abused them, and to support one another. These responses by local faith communities are inspiring, but need to be far more widely replicated.

"Building a new culture of openness and mutual support is essential. Out of this grows the sort of comprehensive change we want to see—change in understandings of masculinity, the end of paralysing stigma, a new approach to legal redress, a place for the leadership and advocacy of survivors themselves, an audible voice for women.

"We sometimes speak of a fivefold response—Prevention, Protection, Provision of services, Prosecution and Partnerships. All I have mentioned so far illustrates how this looks in practice. We are morally and religiously bound to give the highest priority to making this response a universal reality, and are glad to have the support and solidarity of UNAIDS in this. It is a calling that has been laid upon us by a God whose will is always for human dignity and compassion.

"How can UN agencies strengthen their partnership with faith communities to respond more effectively to ending sexual violence?"

Response from Michel Sidibé: "For myself, I make a point of sitting down with religious leaders and faith-based organizations in the countries I visit and talk about ways to partner for people and communities. It is a priority of UNAIDS to engage religious leaders for thoughtful action on critical human rights issues such as sexual violence. In the coming year, I will be traveling to many countries which have high levels of sexual and gender-based violence and mother-to-child transmission of HIV, and will convene with local religious leaders and organizations that are working specifically on these issues. UNAIDS is currently partnering with the Ecumenical Advocacy Alliance, the Global Network of People Living with HIV, and the International Network of Religious Leaders Living with and Affected by HIV to develop a framework for dialogue around HIV. We intend to give religious leaders, people living with HIV, women who have experienced rape, and people most vulnerable to HIV who have been stigmatized greater support and guidance for discussing these difficult issues, hopefully leading to faith community responses like the ones the Archbishop witnessed in

Africa. I am confident that we will all come to greater understanding through this process, and the lives of women, their families and their society will be improved and enriched."[30]

Violence accepted as a norm

The ground realities of the sexual and physical violence that girls and women face are truly frightening. In Ethiopia, for instance, government surveys show that around 23 percent of young girls in the country still undergo the dreadful and harmful practice of female genital mutilation (FGM). According to population surveys, 68.4 percent of Ethiopian women think that wife beating can be justified, and many women are unaware of laws against gender-based violence. As a consequence, few women seek support when facing violence. But these are not unique to Ethiopia.

But it is encouraging to note that the Ethiopian Orthodox Church in Woldia and Kobo, in the northern Amhara region, in collaboration with the UN, has been training hundreds of priests and laity on gender-based violence and is now preaching against violence against women. They are also challenging FGM and are supporting members of school gender clubs. Father Melakesina says, "Many members of the congregation come to me when they have problems. With knowledge on gender-based violence, I intervene and try to prevent it from happening." He continues, "Priests have a major role to play in ending gender-based violence."[31]

Contextual Bible Study and the Tamar Campaign

King David in the Bible is very well known to Christians: the humble shepherd, his success as a king, his lust for Bathsheba, how he plotted and got Uriah (Bathsheba's husband) killed, his repentance, and his heart for worship. However, many have never heard the story about David's daughter, Tamar, an assertive young woman who was raped by her half-brother, Amnon.

In 1996, what started in Pietermaritzburg, South Africa, as a Bible study of Tamar's rape (2 Sam. 13:12-18), by a group of dedicated male and female theologians, developed into a campaign against gender and sexual violence. The Bible study about Tamar's rape disrupts our collective silence on violence against women and brings about transformation and effective solutions. The Tamar Campaign helps churches to address sexual violence and also helps address violent models of masculinity. The campaign was so effective in South Africa that it has spread to other countries within Africa and to other continents.

The Tamar Campaign was created by the Ujamaa Centre for Biblical and Theological Community Development and Research, which is based at the

University of Kwazulu-Natal, Pietermaritzburg. Its primary activities are a series of Bible studies led by trained facilitators. During the Bible study, participants carefully read and analyze the story of Tamar as told in 2 Samuel 13:1-22. They discuss how the passage applies to their own communities, and plan action steps based on what they have learned and discussed. The Bible studies are typically led in churches. While participants spend some time discussing the Bible passage as a large group, they primarily talk in small groups divided by age and gender—older women, younger women, older men, and younger men. To help participants develop their own understandings of the passage, facilitators ask them a series of questions such as:

- What is this text about?

- Who are the male characters and what is the role of each of them in the rape of Tamar?

- What is Tamar's response throughout the story?

- Where is God in this story?

To help participants relate this passage to their own context, facilitators pose additional questions such as, "Are there women like Tamar in your church or community?" "What is the theology of women who have been raped?" and "What message does the story of Tamar have for us?" At the end, facilitators always ask, "What will you now do in response to the Bible study?" and assist with the formulation of action plans. Some churches, for example, have started counselling programs for women in their congregations who have experienced sexual violence, whereas others have hosted workshops that teach men nonviolent ways of expressing their masculinity.

The Tamar Campaign has enabled entire communities to talk about violence against women, but it has especially empowered women whose voices and experiences are often silenced or marginalized within the church. The Tamar Campaign provides an important example of how the Bible can be used as a significant resource for peace, justice, and healing when we integrate biblical theology, communal reflection, and social action. It is also an excellent illustration on how communities of faith can be converted to safe spaces of grace.[32]

The highly acclaimed 2012 WCC-EHAIA publication, *Redemptive Masculinities: Men, HIV, and Religion*, edited by Ezra Chitando and Sophie Chirongoma, strongly asserts that discussion on masculinity in the face of gender-based violence and HIV and AIDS has not taken seriously the role of religion in shaping positive masculine attitudes. Sections of the book also give examples of a theological approach to gender equality and how the traditions and ethics of each of the three major Abrahamic religions can meet the challenge of addressing issues of gender-based violence and HIV and AIDS.[33]

Faith communities carry the great legacy of human endeavour, ingenuity and achievement, diversity, culture, and wisdom through millennia. With the grace of God, we can collectively mobilize this rich experience and legacy to bring about a positive transformation of society. We have to aspire that every congregation is transformed to create safe spaces of grace to deal with the most challenging issues that confront us, as a part of God's household. They must be places where the lonely are welcome; where the trampled find dignity and solace; and where the excluded discover a sacred and safe family and community full of God's grace. Our faith and our foundational values affirm that everyone has a fundamental right to a full life, endowed with good health and well-being!

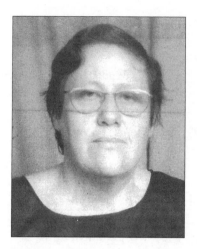

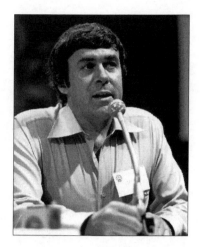

Dr Cecile De Sweemer, deputy
director of the Christian Medical
Commission, WCC (1982–1986)

Rev. Dr David L. Gosling, director
of Church and Society at the WCC

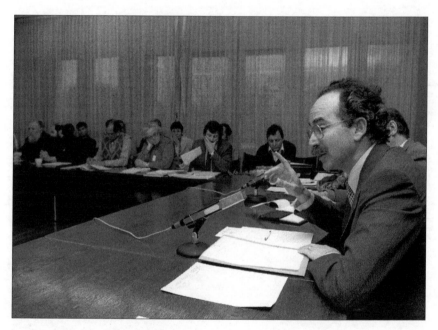

Rev. Dr David L. Gosling, director of Church and Society at the WCC

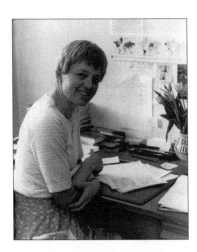

Dr Birgitta Rubenson, the author
of the first WCC resources on HIV
in 1987

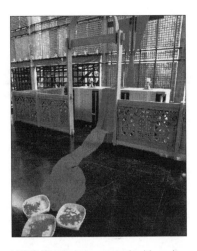

WCC Chapel decorated with red
ribbon for the Central Committee
meeting in 1996

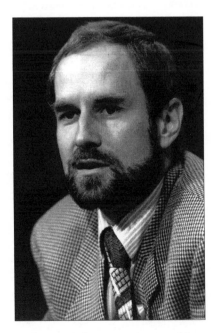

Dr Christoph Benn, moderator of the
WCC consultative group for the study
on HIV and AIDS- 1994 to 1996

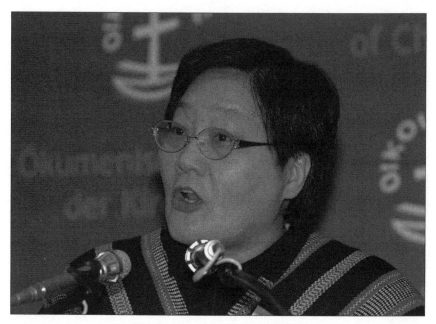

Dr Erlinda Senturias, the Executive Secretary, coordinating the HIV and AIDS
Programme from 1989 to 1997, addressing the WCC's 9th General Assembly in
Porto Alegre, in 2006

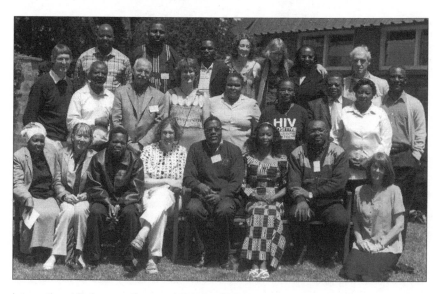

International Reference Group of EHAIA, 2007

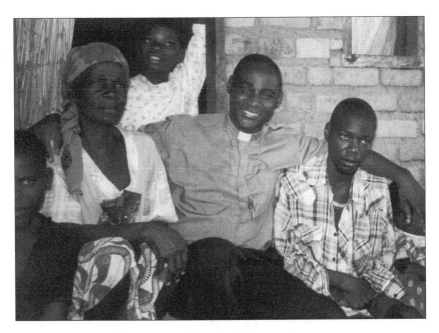

International Reference Group of EHAIA, 2007

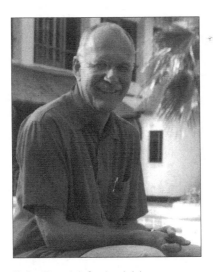

Calle Almedal, Senior Advisor,
UNAIDS, and member if the
International Reference Group -
EHAIA 2002-2008 Photo WCC-EHAIA

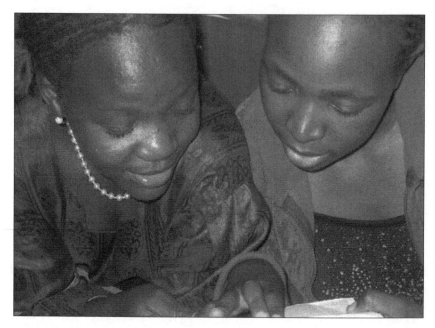

Youth engaged in contextual Bible study, South Africa, 2006. Photo by Dr Sue Parry

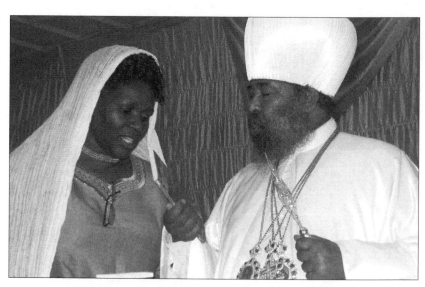

Prof. Musa Dube presenting Prof Ezra Chitando's books, to the late Patriarch of the Ethiopian Orthodox Tewahedo Church, His Holiness Abuna Paulos, in 2008, after a session of Trainer of Trainers for theologians and church leaders on mainstreaming HIV and AIDS. Photo WCC-EHAIA

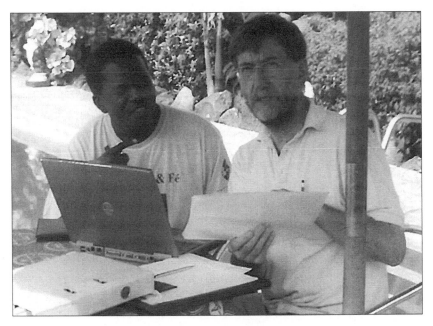

Dr Christoph Mann (r), the first coordinator of EHAIA and Prof. Ezra Chitando, 2006

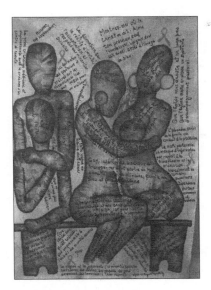

Painting by Ms Essiomle Edinedi, gifted by LGBTIQ groups in Togo, to the General Secretary of the WCC, in recognition of services provided by WCC-EHAIA in West Africa, 2013

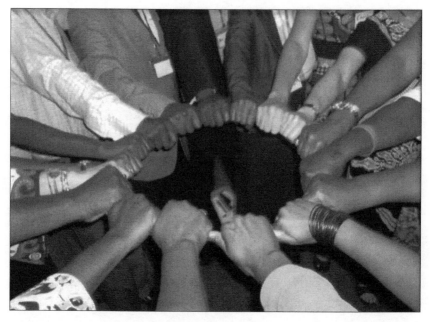

Together, we transform communities! Participants of Council of Churches in Zambia's meeting to review Gender Transformation in Zambian Churches symbolically uniting in action. Photo- PACSA

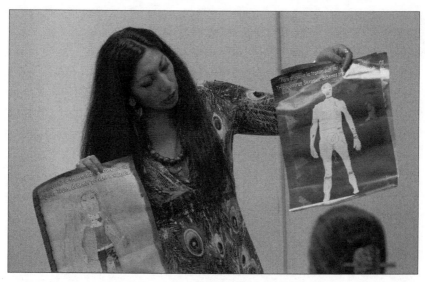

Ms Gracia Violeta conducting a workshop at the Inter-Faith Pre-Conference in Washington, DC, in 2012. Photo by Paul Jeffrey/WCC-EAA

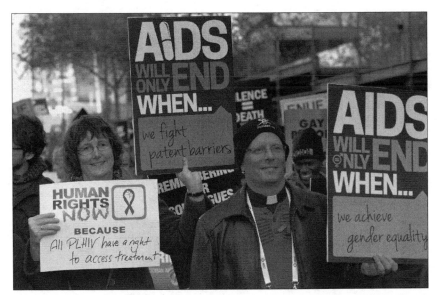

Ms. Astrid Berner-Rodoreda, advisor on HIV and AIDS for Brot für die Welt, and the Rev. Michael Schuenemeyer, executive director of the United Church of Christ HIV and AIDS Network, at a march demanding an end to stigma and discrimination against people living with HIV, held during the 20th International AIDS Conference in Melbourne, Australia, 2014. Photo by Paul Jeffrey for WCC-EAA

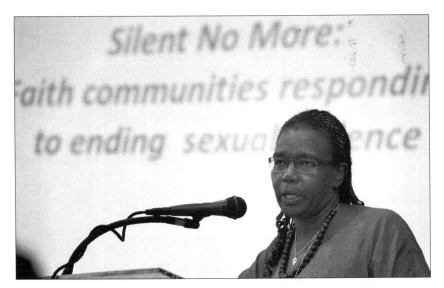

Rev. Dr Nyambura Njoroge, at the "We Will Speak Out" Coalition, which seeks to end sexual violence across communities around the world, an event conducted during the Interfaith Pre-Conference on HIV, 2012 in Washington, DC. Photo by Paul Jeffrey/WCC-EAA

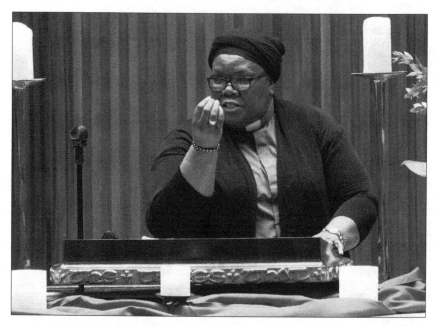

Rev Phumzile Mabizela, executive director of the International Network of Religious Leaders Living with or Personally Affected by HIV or AIDS (INERELA+), at the 2016 High-Level Meeting on Ending AIDS Interfaith Prayer Service, 7 June 2016, at the United Nations Church Center in New York.

Chapter 5

Walk the Walk, Talk the Talk

"By this everyone will know that you are my disciples,
if you have love for one another."—John 13:35

The discussions that took the form of a "dialogue" in the 1970s between Dr John H. Bryant, the WCC's Christian Commission's chairman and a professor of public health, and Rev. David E. Jenkins, a commission member and a theologian, brought to the forefront the greatest challenges that society faces and how these can be dealt with morally and ethically. Although both approached the challenges from different points of view, both were committed to a distribution of resources that improved the lot of those worst off. Bryant addressed the question of "healthcare and justice," applying the notions of entitlement, natural rights, positive rights, and distributive justice to the question of human health. Jenkins approached the question differently. For him, the Bible is concerned about "human possibilities, about divine activities, and about human response to divine activities" and with "obstacles to becoming human." Consequently, it is much more concerned with "attacking exploitations, attacking oppressions, attacking inequalities, attacking deprivation than laying down rights."[1]

It is very clear from the discussions that we not only have to be technically competent to deal with current-day challenges.[2] We also have to be ethically and morally rooted to live with the problems that confront our society. As people of faith, we have to be present on the ground, accompanying people through the daily challenges. In this chapter, I offer different narratives about and from the ecumenical movement's co-workers to show how they are walking the walk and talking the talk in seven key areas of engagement.

Accompaniment

In his book *Living with Hope*,[3] Ezra Chitando describes accompaniment in a very touching and effective manner:

> Among the Shona people of Zimbabwe, as with other African cultural groups, visitors are to be treated with utmost courtesy. When visitors announce their departure, hosts are expected to try to persuade them to stay. When visitors leave, hosts are expected to see them out of the homestead. More importantly, they are also expected to travel with them for a good part of the journey. *Kuperekedza* (to accompany) implies identifying with the person undertaking a journey. In effect, they are told, "You are not alone on this journey. I share your struggle." Churches are called upon to live out the positive attitude towards travellers that is found in African societies. It must express solidarity with people living with HIV. It must engage in accompaniment. It must travel with people living with HIV and be sensitive to their rights and needs. Crucially, it must break down barriers between "us" and "them." A church "with friendly feet" walks alongside those affected by HIV. It courageously proclaims that it is a church living with HIV and AIDS. It refuses to throw stones (John 8:1–11) and recognizes that the gospel compels Christians to love without limits. As it accompanies people and communities living with HIV and AIDS on journeys of faith, the church with friendly feet ministers to every need. It repents of its negative attitudes, as well as the stigma and discrimination surrounding the disease. As it works with and among those living with HIV, it interrogates its theology, its attitude to sexuality and its gender insensitivity. It awakens to the realization that it must become an all-embracing community. A church with friendly feet does not pose questions about the moral standing of those with whom it is journeying.

The ecumenical movement has been quite strong on this dimension of the HIV ministry. Since its inception, WCC-EHAIA has played an effective role in journeying with different categories of activists in its response to HIV and AIDS. In the previous chapter, reference was made to the role that WCC-EHAIA has played in engaging theological institutions to mainstream HIV in their curricula. Alongside WCC-EHAIA, other ecumenical networks focusing on research and publication in theology and HIV emerged. These include the African Network of Higher Education and Research in Religion, Theology, HIV and AIDS (ANERTHA) and the Collaborative for HIV and AIDS, Religion and Theology (CHART) in South Africa.

WCC-EHAIA has also accompanied groups of young people living with HIV, such as Youth Engage, in Zimbabwe and in Togo. In addition, WCC-EHAIA has journeyed with networks of women living with HIV, same-sex-loving individuals and groups, as well as groups of people with disability. The operative words in these ecumenical engagements have been *solidarity, accompaniment,* and *upholding justice* and *human dignity.*

WCC-EHAIA's Contribution in Transformative Masculinity—Prof. Ezra Chitando

WCC-EHAIA's work on transformative masculinity has generated immense interest within the faith communities and beyond. In Nigeria, it has promoted interfaith dialogue on what it means to be men who profess to be Christian or Muslim, and how this relates to acting for peace and social transformation. In 2015, workshops were held in different Nigerian settings on how Christians and Muslims could draw on the positive values of masculinity within the two traditions. When this is combined with the quest for transformative masculinity within African indigenous cultures, it provides the foundation for more peaceful, tolerant, and loving ways of being male in contexts of religious bigotry, sexual and gender-based violence, and HIV.

In Namibia, partnership has been deepened with the White Ribbon Campaign. Using the resource of Contextual Bible Study, participants to WCC-EHAIA's White Ribbon Campaign workshops have explored the positive role of the Bible in shaping new models of being male. In Lesotho, the "Transformative Masculinity" campaign has extended beyond the faith communities into the correctional services. By partnering with the uniformed services, WCC-EHAIA has succeeded in raising awareness of the dangers of toxic definitions of masculinity and the need to generate redemptive masculinities. In Botswana, "Transformative Masculinity" workshops across the years have led to the formation of a men's movement, the Pitso Ya Banna Association. This represents a deepening of the transformative masculinity concept as the men in Botswana have expressed their commitment to continuing with the work in their local and national contexts. Transformative masculinity concepts have also been popular in Madagascar, Zimbabwe, Malawi, and other countries.

One of the most notable successes of WCC-EHAIA's work with boys and men has been to challenge men to appreciate the cost of hegemonic masculinity to men's very own health and well-being. This has mobilized men to seek change in the religious, social, cultural, economic, and political spheres from the position of enlightened self-interest. Men are still challenged to work in solidarity with girls and women, but they would have already "bought into" the need for gender justice. Transformative masculinity represents one of the most innovative and liberating concepts that has emerged in the ecumenical movement's engagement with HIV and AIDS in the recent past.

Accompanying Children

Virginia's story, narrated by Rev. Pauline Wanjiru Njiru

We discovered Virginia through her grandmother, who told us how sad she was for her granddaughter who had completed secondary school successfully and was eligible to join university but, due to lack of support, had disappeared and her whereabouts were unknown. By the time we found her in 2012, she was married with two children. She was excited at the thought of joining the university and she gave it her best shot. Virginia Wanjiru now holds a degree from the St Paul's University, thanks to the support that was mobilized from the United Church of Canada, and the guidance of Prof. Esther Mombo and Dr Nyambura Njoroge. Just before her graduation in 2015, she wrote:

> Being brought up by my grandmother together with my two brothers in Mai-Mahiu village life was not easy. My grandmother had to work very hard to make sure that everything was well with us. Despite my absence after my o-level she still had a heart and a vision I go on with my studies. Through God's mercy, my grandmother's prayers, and people like you who were willing to support me, the opportunity to study I thought had vanished was realized. I am the first person in my family to attend university, and I hope to set a fine example for my younger brother, cousins, and friends in the village. My future career plans include enrolling for CPA courses in January next year, pursuing a masters in operation research and a PhD in risk management. I not only have a passion for auditing, but also a vision to help make my community more developed with the skill that I have acquired in the university. Rev. Pauline always supported me, gave me hope by watching, listening, and wiping my tears whenever I felt lonely and she become my role model a mother and a friend.

Consolata Ng'endo

Consolata Ng'endo was 14 years old when we met her, assisting her paralyzed mother living with HIV, at a one-day seminar organized by the Nyakandu disability group that we were invited to facilitate. Consolata was neglected and unkempt, with little support of facilities to maintain herself and her mother. They were living in deplorable conditions in a swamp and she had fallen behind in her studies. She was in in grade five, while her peers were in grade ten. Consolata described her life as an ordeal: at 15 she was the breadwinner, and she would either work or beg for food to feed her two dependents and earn money to take her mother to the clinic. She had repeated the same class for many years since she missed out on school many times and especially during her menstrual periods, as she could not afford sanitary towels.

We invited Consolata to the November consultation in Nairobi in 2015. Her confidence was unmatched as she expressed herself in broken English and sometimes vernacular. We engaged the Nyakandu disability group, which is a merry-go-round group of people living with HIV, people with disability, and people with both, who agreed to look after Consolata's mother while Consolata pursued her dream to get an education. My two friends and I initialized this arrangement from our personal resources and got her to a boarding school. She is happy and vibrant, and her mother and little brother are also doing well, so we hope that Consolata will get a sponsor, too.

Sunday School Teachers and Chaplains Workshop on "New Strategies of Prevention and HIV"—Ayoko Bahun-Wilson

From 24 to 26 February 2016 in Lomé, Togo, the WCC-EHAIA West Africa Regional Office organized a two-day meeting for 25 Sunday school teachers and chaplains from various denominations such as the Methodist Church of Togo, the Evangelical Presbyterian Church of Togo, the Assemblies of God, the Baptist Convention, and the Pentecostal Church around the theme "New strategies of prevention and HIV."

The workshop, fully organized and funded by WCC-EHAIA, aimed at raising the awareness of the new preventive methods and particularly defining new approaches to reach out to the adolescents and youth. Teachers and chaplains during the two days reflected on how they could holistically reach out to children and ensure that they had all the needed information on their adolescence and be able to make positive choices.

The various themes discussed—such as HIV prevention in schools and its challenges; sexuality, violence, and HIV infection in juvenile environments; roles of Sunday school teachers and chaplains in the HIV response—were intended to reach out to teens by providing in-depth knowledge of the challenges that they face, as statistics show that adolescents are now the most affected.

Young-girl education continues to be a challenge, as the rate of early pregnancies in primary and secondary schools is very high. In Togo, not only are teens are being infected by HIV but also many early pregnancies are being recorded. 2013 statistics indicated that, nationally, 86 percent of girls had access to primary school but only 29 percent reached secondary schools, while 72 percent of boys continued their schooling. In the six regions in Togo, between 2010 and 2012, out of 5443 pregnancies, 230 were recorded from primary schools.[4] These statistics invite Sunday school teachers to reflect on their roles and help adolescents and young people to protect themselves. Among the many preoccupations of delegates during the two days, the main one was, "Is the family still a safe space for the young girl, as it seems that it has failed in its role of prime educator of the girl vis-à-vis her sexual and reproductive health?"

Chaplains and Sunday school teachers should aim at transforming the weaknesses of adolescents and youth to strengths to be able to respond appropriately to their challenges. Chaplaincies, which are more and more marginalized today when they are meant to be the epicenter where adolescents and young people from churches find solace, have been again identified as places where action can be taken in times of stress and wrong attitudes. They should be considered as key places where churches can develop strategies and solutions to some challenges. A chaplain from the Evangelical Presbyterian Church of Togo, Rev. Amedodji Etienne, said, "If as Sunday school teachers and chaplains, we are able to save one child, it is a whole population who is saved."

Contextual Bible Study has helped participants to create a safe space to discuss the situations of adolescents and youths in a situation of violence. The case of Tamar in 2 Samuel 13:1-22, and the experience of Zouhoura, the young girl from Chad who was raped on 13 February 2016 by a gang of five young boys, created a rich debate on measures to take to prevent such violence in the society and the church.

To conclude, a pastor from the Pentecostal Church of Togo, Rev. Dakla Komla, said: "Today children are born digital and therefore need digital parents and not analogical; this will help build a strong relationship between parents and children." The workshop ended on a positive note, with leaders committed to taking action in churches and schools, both public and private, to raise the alarm on the importance of comprehensive education on sex, violence, and HIV. As an immediate action, one delegate is planning a day-long programme for 500 adolescents from primary schools in Lomé.

Accompanying Young Women

Stand up, speak out!—Vanessa R. Anyoti, Programmes Associate and Young Women's Program Coordinator, World YWCA

I never quite fully understood the notion that faith can be a liberating force for girls and women. The actuality is that there exist "life-giving texts which affirm that all human beings are created in the image of God." (Okondo, SRHR and Rights for Young Women).

Since its implementation in 2008, the Tamar Campaign has done just that. In the YWCA of Mwanza branch, located in the lake zone of Tanzania, I was able to see how a Contextual Bible Study (CBS) group, which meets on a monthly basis, was actively influencing the community. This CBS group not only consisted of people from different faiths but also a majority of women living with HIV and AIDS. To me, this opened my eyes to the way CBS can be a unifying force among people of different faiths, providing hope and comfort for women, young women, and men afflicted by grief. Why? Because the CBS provides a basis to recognize the true essence of a human being and thus value equality of all peoples. Now, the group has gone further and is looking at entrepreneurial measures as well as local saving and investment groups that it can establish to economically empower its members. That to me is the description of faith, love, and equality. The Tamar Campaign has put this in action.

This foundation, based on the equality of all peoples, is the footing that dreams and development flourish on. As a young woman, it is clear to me that gender inequality, discrimination, stigma, the failure to fully realize the rights of others, and the like are due to the fact that we do not view others as equal to ourselves. We thus, knowingly or unknowing, perpetuate such acts as violence. I can also attest to the influence faith has, both positive and negative, on my peers and others. Faith has hindered people on matters such as advocacy regarding violence against women and girls (VAW/g); the reporting of cases to legal authorities; follow through on legal cases; reconciliation; and the provision of holistic mental and physical services, and the like. Through Tamar, young people are taking center stage and challenging these notions by conducting community outreach, working with religious leaders, and providing legal services to address VAW/g. We believe that, if we can uplift young women, and promote the notion of equality, then we can actively and whole-heartedly participate in change and development.

Stand up, speak out, and seek justice, because you and I are equal!

Accompanying LGBTIQ

Faith communities in the context of human sexuality—Ayoko Bahun-Wilson, West Africa

In Togo, the LGBTIQ associations have been accompanied since 2012 and have received in various ways the support of WCC-EHAIA. Often, WCC-EHAIA is being asked to provide technical assistance during the organization of workshops and to break the silence on issues of stigma, discrimination, homophobia, and family mediation. WCC-EHAIA has forged strategic links with National Aids Commissions in different countries in West Africa and with Family Health International 360 (FHI 360) on joint efforts for the integration of LGBTIQ in the various programmes. The support WCC-EHAIA provided to help ensure a well-equipped LGBTIQ drop-in center, first created in Lomé by FHI 360, is a visible example. WCC-EHAIA uses Contextual Bible Study in its training workshops to raise the awareness of religious leaders on the reality of the LGBTIQ group. In Benin, in 2014, the Protestant University in West Africa organized an interdisciplinary conference on LGBTIQ issues, where lecturers and students were exposed to the reality of LGBTIQ persons and engaged in in-depth reflection on how they could respond appropriately to that reality in their various settings when they went back to their settings. In Nigeria, the Faculty of Social Sciences of the State University of Ibadan is doing a research project on sexual diversity with the support of WCC-EHAIA, while in Togo, in 2015, the Faculty of Humanities of the University of Lomé published, with WCC-EHAIA assistance, a book on *Body, Masculinity, Femininity and HIV.* Another visible sign of accompaniment provided to the LGBTIQ group is the process that led to the gift of a painting done by Ms. Essiomle Edinedi, which was handed over to the General Secretary of the WCC in his Geneva office in 2013.

Members who participated in the WCC-EHAIA workshops have enjoyed the themes developed, which has had an impact on some aspects of their attitudes and their views on key populations. A Catholic participant testified: "I had chased from home a family member who was homosexual, but since that training I apologized and asked him to return home. I now look at him like a child of God with his sexual orientation." The same person continued and said the following about street children: "After the training, I had the courage to approach them and discuss their future with them. I even managed to persuade two of them to start trading. They are no longer on the street and have now built a hut in the compound." These children also realized changes in their attitude about homosexuality: "The discussion on homosexuality and key populations was difficult to be accepted by our relations but are now easier, especially when we talk to them about the likelihood that men who have sex with men [MSM] are a bridge population in the transmission of HIV infection." Again, on homosexuality another said: "For me, homosexuality did not exist. But after this training, I became aware of that sexual orientation and I'm prepared to understand and accept in order to help if they are infected and thus help break the chain of transmission."

Another participant said, "This workshop has helped me personally to be reassured about my Christian faith because I could get answers to the questions I was asking myself, [such as,] "Can a professional sex worker go to church on Sundays? Can she/he pay his/her tithe knowing the origin of the money?" Regular feedback workshops are being held with her colleague sex workers and some of them "began attending church on Sundays, convinced that they will not be judged and that pastors will help them to be tolerated as children of God." One Moro Naaba gave this testimony: "I was in the army and the secret service and I used to be placed in prisons just to identify MSM and ensured that they are never set free because of their orientation. I thought that was the best way to get rid of them, but now with this new insight from this workshop, I realise that MSM are also human beings created in the image of God and I will share this knowledge with my colleagues to stop that practice."[5]

Accompanying Interfaith Programmes on HIV and AIDS

AINA and other Asian efforts—Erlinda N. Senturias

Religion and faith have played a major role in the history of humankind. In the midst of suffering and misery, religious leaders have played significant roles in alleviating suffering and creating new communities of love, compassion, and understanding. Their response to HIV and AIDS should be no different. Many ancient cultures and religions have been born in the crucible of Asia, gifting to the world a rich heritage of philosophical and religious thinking.

The work on HIV and AIDS by the interfaith communities did not start when everyone in our faith communities were ready to do the work on HIV. Some religious leaders faced rejection in their own communities when they started to work with people living with HIV. We started with a few committed religious leaders who were already accompanying people on the ground and who were also looking for solidarity with other religious leaders, as it was not fashionable to do work on AIDS in the early years of 1990.

Two of the greatest supporters of the HIV program were Rev. Prawate Khid-arn, then General Secretary of the Christian Conference of Asia, and the

Venerable Phra Maha Boonchuay Doojai of the Buddhist faith tradition. Both became chairpersons of the Asian Interfaith Network on AIDS (AINA). Venerable Phra Maha Boonchuay Doojai said, "as a Buddhist monk in Thailand, it is difficult to collaborate with other faiths in many areas, but my personal interest and commitment to foster good relations with other faiths is the reason to work in this area." His active involvement on HIV and AIDS opened the doors of Buddhist communities for us to see and interact with them on the Buddhist program initiatives not only in Thailand but also in our relations with religious leaders in other countries in Asia.

On the other hand, Rev. Prawate Khid-arn was accompanied in his work by the Church of Christ in Thailand AIDS Ministry, led by Rev. Sanan Wutti and his team of pastors, who are supporting people living with HIV and AIDS in Thailand. In fact, their work on HIV gave me much inspiration and passion for the work on HIV in the World Council of Churches since 1990.

In 2001, a dialogue for the creation of an Asian Interfaith Network on HIV and AIDS (AINA) in Thailand organized by the Christian Conference of Asia was followed by a subregional consultation of church leaders of South Asian Churches in Colombo in July 2002 and two interfaith AIDS conferences organized in Bangkok in the years 2003 and 2004. These brought together Buddhist, Christian, Hindu, and Muslim representatives and, in May 2005, AINA was formally launched regionally in Chiang Mai, culminating in a steering committee of ten people representing different faiths and people living with HIV and AIDS. AINA's mission was the building of caring communities, ensuring the promotion and protection of human rights, with support from governmental and nongovernmental agencies, international organizations, and multisectoral organizations whenever necessary. Its program and activities include the study and research of the interface between faiths and the AIDS epidemic; disseminating information through a newsletter and electronic network; capacity building in training and personnel exchange; and campaigning on critical issues, because AINA believes in the greater involvement of people living with HIV and AIDS in all programmes and activities.

AINA connects and supports Christian, Muslim, Hindu, and Buddhist religious leaders in the fight against HIV and AIDS. AINA's objectives are to establish and promote country-level interfaith HIV and AIDS networks, to build the capacity of faith-based organizations in responding to the epidemic, and to create a supportive environment for faith-based responses to HIV and AIDS. The network focuses on the fight against all forms of discrimination against people living with HIV and AIDS and those affected by it. Today, AINA members hail from Thailand, India, Myanmar, Vietnam, Laos, Cambodia, Sri Lanka, Bangladesh, Indonesia, and Korea.

During my time as HIV consultant with the Christian Conference of Asia, one of the countries where I did the accompanying work of building an interfaith network was in Myanmar. I was present in the establishment of the Myanmar Interfaith Network on HIV and AIDS (MINA) in May 2009. Through our connection with MINA, we had been blessed with the participation of seven networks (Myanmar Positive Group, Myanmar Positive Women Network, MSM Network, Sex Workers in Myanmar [SWIM], National Drug Users Network, and the National NGO Network, where MINA became an active participant). The Myanmar Positive Christian Network and religious leaders who are living with HIV and AIDS also shared their precious stories to the group who came for the roundtable on HIV in Yangon, Myanmar, in June 2011.

The participants read the pledge of commitment developed for the religious leaders by the Ecumenical Advocacy Alliance (now the WCC Ecumenical Advocacy Alliance) and owned it as their own pledge, promising to ensure zero stigma and discrimination of people living with HIV and AIDS, zero gender-based violence, and zero new HIV infections in their interfaith network.

The presence of the members of the Asian Interfaith Network on AIDS (AINA) like the Indian Interfaith Coalition on AIDS (IICA), the Indonesian Interfaith Network on AIDS (INTERNA), and the Interfaith Network on HIV and AIDS in Thailand (INHAT) encouraged the other countries to set up their own interfaith networks like Bangladesh. A significant development was also the formation of the Singapore Interfaith Network on AIDS (SINA) through our connection with Bishop Yap Kim Hao, former General Secretary of the Christian Conference of Asia in the early 1970s. At 83 years old, he is actively providing accompaniment to marginalized communities like the gay church and sex workers network in Singapore. He is also helping people living with HIV to have access to medicines from the health ministry of Singapore. We became closer following the Christian Conference of Asia General Assembly in Kuala Lumpur in 2010 when we attended a worship service in that city's gay church. At the pre-assembly conference, jointly sponsored with the Christian Conference of Asia and Ecumenical Advocacy Alliance, AINA agreed to develop additional training resources to help religious leaders and FBOs better combat stigma and discrimination against those affected by HIV and AIDS.

AINA holds interfaith pre-activities during the International Conference on AIDS in Asia and the Pacific. The last that I accompanied as a staff member of the Christian Conference of Asia was the meeting that was held in Busan, Korea, in August 2011, where the Korean Interfaith Network on AIDS was formed and actively joined us in the follow-up meeting in Siem Reap to make strategic plans for the interfaith work on HIV and AIDS. This was reported during the interfaith conference meetings during the International Conference on AIDS in Asia and the Pacific in Bangkok, Thailand, in November 2011.

Comprehensive HIV Care

Faith-based provision of health services has been a cornerstone of the global response to HIV from the earliest days of the HIV and AIDS epidemic. Africa, which has 10 percent of the world's population, but 25 percent of the global disease burden, is home to nearly a third of all people living with HIV and AIDS, with some countries in Southern Africa having HIV prevalence rates above 20 percent. In this context, faith-based healthcare providers deliver a large proportion of comprehensive HIV care to millions of people on a daily basis. With their holistic engagement and collaboration with communities, they can ensure effective biomedical responses to epidemics and health emergencies. But it has to be noted that many faith-based health services work under severe constraints, especially regarding their workforce.[6] This heroic role of health professionals on the frontlines of dealing with epidemics is further evidenced by the fact that a significant proportion of the more than 200 doctors, nurses, and other healthcare workers who have died of Ebola since June 2014 worked in hospitals and health centres run by churches.

In 2012, Ambassador Eric Goosby, who served as the United States Global AIDS Coordinator from 2009 until mid-November 2013, directed the U.S. strategy for addressing HIV around the world, and led President Obama's implementation of the President's Emergency Plan for AIDS Relief (PEPFAR), acknowledged that

> Without the contributions of our faith-based organization (FBO) partners, the U.S. President's Emergency Plan for AIDS Relief (PEPFAR) could not have achieved the extraordinary impact on the HIV/AIDS epidemic of the past decade. Supporting antiretroviral treatment for nearly 4 million people living with HIV, interventions to prevent mother-to-child transmission that allowed approximately 200,000 infants to be born HIV-free in 2011 alone, care for over 4 million orphans and vulnerable children—FBOs have been central to all of these achievements. These partners work with us in areas of the world that have been hardest hit by AIDS. In sub-Saharan Africa, it is estimated that 40 percent of health care services are provided by FBOs, many of which serve the most rural areas and the most marginalized people. FBOs have long histories

and strong community roots, and a deep reservoir of trust on which to draw. Robust participation of FBOs is not optional—it is essential for an effective response to AIDS.[7]

Key Ecumenical Partners

The Catholic Church (which is a partner of the WCC and closely works with others in the ecumenical movement) is one of the biggest global health providers. It runs thousands of hospitals and dispensaries as well as houses for people who are elderly, chronically ill, or who have physical or learning disabilities.

Caritas Internationalis (which translates as "love between peoples") is the official diaconal arm of the Catholic Church and consists of more than 160 national members. Caritas works to provide healthcare in emergencies where people are vulnerable to illness and disease. Teams from national Caritas organizations quickly set up temporary clinics to treat water-borne infections and eye, skin, and chest conditions. They provide information and supplies to prevent illness from spreading. Caritas supports the existing medical services, which may be in danger of being overwhelmed by the crisis. When there is no emergency, Caritas seeks to keep people in good health, especially the most poor and vulnerable. This means running clinics, dispensaries, and screening, prevention, and treatment programmes around the world.

Since 1987, Caritas has prioritized efforts in response to the pandemic of HIV and AIDS. More than 100 members of the Caritas Confederation are engaged in providing value-based prevention education, treatment, care, and support to people living with or affected by HIV in all parts of the world. It advocates with governments, international organizations, and drug companies for universal access to cost-effective and suitable medicines.[8]

World Vision, which is also a key ecumenical partner, reaches 1 million orphans and children made vulnerable by AIDS each year. World Vision trains and mobilizes thousands of community members through CCCs to provide care for orphans and vulnerable children and people living with HIV. They also run Channels of Hope, which, through experiential workshops and follow-up, equips faith leaders to reduce HIV-related stigma in their communities and promote compassionate care for people and families affected by HIV. These workshops have reached more than 150,000 faith leaders.[9]

While specialized health services, and the professionals needed to run them, remain an integral part of Christian mission in many parts of the world, the local congregation's participation in the healing mission of the church is a major part of the continuum of professional care that the churches and the ecumenical partners provide.

Advocacy

The ecumenical movement has been very active in the international arena, lifting up the voices of communities and the people served by churches. A very visible example has been the work of the WCC-Ecumenical Advocacy Alliance (WCC-EAA), which was initiated by an international network of churches and church-related organizations committed to campaigning together on common concerns. HIV and AIDS was chosen as one of the two pressing issues around which to do global advocacy. HIV remains one of the two campaigns to date. The WCC-EAA has been organizing interfaith pre-conferences associated with every International AIDS Conferences since 2004. These conferences are held every two years, and draw over 20,000 researchers, policymakers, activists, people living with HIV, and others to share the latest advances and to help identify and tackle continued obstacles to the pandemic. The WCC-EAA weaves deep spirituality, prayer, and worship into both the pre-conference and the main conference, in addition to organizing the conference chaplaincy services. The prayers services organized at these conferences bring together faith communities from different religions and denominations, and consolidate their commitment to international advocacy. The liturgies that are developed each year for the World AIDS Day on 1 December are widely used all over the world.

The work of the WCC-EAA in advocating for access to medication has also been significant. The campaign for increasing access to pediatric HIV medication has been carried out to take action to help children living with HIV. An action guide, called "Prescription for Life," encourages young people around the world to take action to help children living with HIV. The guide provides information and resources for schools, families, faith groups, and communities to empower young people in writing letters to pharmaceutical companies and governments to improve testing and treatment for infants and children living with HIV. WCC-EAA also continues to advocate for better access to second- and third-line treatments, especially in lower- to middle-income countries.

The WCC-EAA also has been coordinating ecumenical engagement on the issue of HIV at the United Nations, in preparation for the High-Level Meeting (HLM) of the United Nations General Assembly scheduled to take place in New York, 8–10 June 2016. The HLM will undertake a comprehensive review of the progress achieved in realizing the 2001 Declaration of Commitment on HIV/AIDS and the 2006 and 2011 Political Declaration on HIV/AIDS. The WCC-EAA has set up an HLM planning working group to strategize and coordinate the advocacy activities for the High-Level Meeting. In addition, HIV Campaign Coordinator Francesca Merico and campaign strategy group member Stuart

Kean (from World Vision) are members of the Civil Society Advisory Group, which is drafting the Civil Society Outcome Document for the HLM.

The WCC-EAA also assists churches in confronting the reality that, even after such an eventful ecumenical journey with HIV, people around the world living with HIV still endure assaults on their dignity and basic human rights— from stigma and discrimination to denial of legal protection and even medical care. As part of this endeavour, with the support of the Norwegian Agency for Development Cooperation (NORAD) and UNAIDS, the WCC recently published a significant book titled *Dignity, Freedom, and Grace: Christian Perspectives on HIV, AIDS, and Human Rights*. This thought-provoking and challenging publication brings together 23 contributors' insights and reflections—always lively, sometimes uncomfortable, often deeply moving—that search for common ground in combatting HIV.[10]

The other vital advocacy campaign that has deep implications for overcoming AIDS is "Thursdays in Black," a campaign against sexual and gender-based violence. Thursdays in Black was started by the WCC in the 1980s as a form of peaceful protest against rape and violence, especially that which takes place during wars and conflicts. The campaign focuses on ways by which individuals may challenge attitudes that cause rape and violence. The Thursdays in Black campaign was faithfully observed in South Africa by the Diakonia Council of Churches and the Christian AIDS Bureau of Southern Africa (CABSA), ecumenical partners of the WCC's project Ecumenical HIV and AIDS Initiative in Africa (WCC-EHAIA) and the International Network of Religious Leaders Living with or Personally Affected by HIV or AIDS (INERELA+). After its 10th assembly in Busan, Republic of Korea, the WCC is working with its partner organizations to revive the Thursdays in Black campaign. Partners include CABSA, We Will Speak Out Coalition, the Lutheran World Federation, the Fellowship of the Least Coin, the United Methodist Women, and the World YWCA, among others.

The Christian understanding of health, healing, and the healing ministry is related to the Christian understanding of salvation and the realization of the reign of God. This realization is the "new creation" that the biblical prophets announced and anticipated as "shalom." Shalom can be described as an ultimate state of reconciled and healed relationships between creation and God, between humanity and God, humanity and creation, and between humans as individuals and as groups or societies. Each act of accompaniment and healing is a sign of the realization of shalom.

Chapter 6

Visions of the Future

The End of AIDS Is on the Horizon and within Our Grasp

Since the early days of the AIDS epidemic, in 1983, the world has come a long way. Now, we have the knowledge and the tools to end AIDS. Although we see the tantalizing vision of ending the HIV epidemic on the horizon, there are real risks for the journey ahead and there is no room for complacency. In this concluding chapter, I offer an overview of the risks and possibilities and some key insights we have learned from dealing with HIV, which will equip us to deal with many other social and public-health challenges we face today and perhaps face in the future.

Comprehensive HIV care

With 37 million HIV-positive people and more than two million new infections annually, HIV remains a major world health challenge. But there has been rapid progress in treating HIV, and now over 15 million people are accessing antiretroviral therapy (ART). Evidence shows the amazing advances in the clinical care of HIV-affected patients after the adoption of potent ART.[1] The many efficacious drug combinations available today can recover the immune system even in patients presenting at a very advanced stage. In high-income countries, 90 percent of patients who adhere to ART can achieve full HIV suppression. In resource-limited settings, especially in countries where free ART programmes have been implemented, similar trends have been demonstrated. It is estimated that worldwide mortality declined by 35 percent from 2005 to 2013.[2] In December 2014, UNAIDS announced that taking a "fast-track approach" over the next five years will allow the world to end the AIDS epidemic by 2030. It is estimated that this fast-track approach would avert nearly 28 million new HIV infections and 21 million AIDS-related deaths by 2030. To achieve this goal, a new set of targets would need to be reached by 2020. This includes achieving 90–90–90: 90 percent of people living with HIV knowing their HIV status; 90 percent of people who know their HIV-positive status on treatment; and 90 percent of people on treatment with suppressed viral loads.[3]

The modelling exercise supporting the 90–90–90 strategy predicts that at least 73 percent of the entire viral load of all HIV-positive individuals must be suppressed (a very low level of HIV in the body) to have a substantial effect on HIV transmission at a population level.[4] Unfortunately, even data on the "HIV treatment cascade"[5] (or the HIV care continuum) from the best centres shows only around 35 percent of the overall HIV population is fully suppressed. In the USA, the Centers for Disease Control and Prevention estimate that only 25 percent of HIV-positive people are suppressed. This implies that for the world to achieve the end of AIDS, the sequential steps or stages of HIV medical care that people living with HIV go through—from diagnosis of HIV infection, linkage to care, retention in care, receipt of antiretroviral therapy, and achievement of viral suppression—has to be very efficient. Therefore, complacency at any stage could jeopardize the progress so far. Countries with weaker health systems must be empowered to do their utmost to ensure that comprehensive care for people living with HIV is protected from disruption. Until there is a cure, HIV infection must be prevented from progressing to AIDS by providing patients with accessible, consistent, and reliable care. Comprehensive HIV care also implies the availability and access of proven interventions, namely: screening the blood supply, availability of condoms, provision of education for behaviour modification, HIV testing and counselling, treatment/prevention of drug and alcohol abuse, providing clean syringes, antiretrovirals (ARVs) to prevent mother-to-child transmission of HIV, post-exposure prophylaxis against HIV by using ART, male circumcision, treatment of other sexually transmitted infections, and pre-exposure prophylaxis against HIV by using ARVs.

The UNAIDS report *Fast-Track: Ending the AIDS Epidemic by 2030* also highlights how critical investment is to achieve these targets. Low-income countries will require a peak of US $9.7 billion in funding in 2020 and lower-middle-income countries US $8.7 billion. International funding support will be needed to supplement domestic investments, particularly in low-income countries, which are currently funding only around 10 percent of their responses to HIV through domestic sources. Upper-middle-income countries will require US $17.2 billion in 2020. In 2013, 80 percent of upper-middle-income countries were financing their responses to HIV through domestic sources.[6]

Nine countries in sub-Saharan Africa (Ethiopia, Kenya, Malawi, Nigeria, South Africa, Tanzania, Uganda, Zambia, and Zimbabwe) account for 70 percent of the burden of HIV and AIDS in Africa. A new modelling study suggests there is a significant shortfall in the funding that these countries will need in order to control the disease in the years to come.

In the March 2016 *BMJ Open* journal, researchers at Harvard University's T. H. Chan School of Public Health in Cambridge, Massachusetts, estimate the funding that the nine sub-Sahara African countries will need to treat and prevent HIV between 2015 and 2050. The model calculates a significant shortfall between financing obligations and future funding available, showing that none of the countries can meet future obligations.[7] The first author, Rifat Atun, professor of global health systems at Harvard University, says: "The HIV epidemic is far from over. The magnitude of funding needed to sustain the HIV fight is very large and the consequences of complacency even larger." Professor Atun and colleagues say "front-loading"[8] investments are needed to secure the higher levels of coverage required to ultimately reduce HIV spread. Such up-front investment will also reduce future funding obligations. They note that new, innovative sources of finance must be sought to maintain and expand HIV treatment and prevention, as domestic financing—currently the main source of funding—will not be enough.[9]

Dr Stefano Vella, from Istituto Superiore di Sanità, and the past president of the International AIDS Society, in his 2015 article in *The Lancet HIV*, "End of AIDS on the Horizon, but Innovation Needed to End HIV," cautions us that "AIDS is indeed more manageable everywhere. But the HIV epidemic is definitely not over. Let's not leave the job half-done!"[10]

Vulnerability, justice, and compassion

We can compare the journey to overcome HIV to an epic marathon race, each year representing a kilometre, for a total of forty-two. We have made it to the 34th year and have approached the last and the most testing stretch. The greatest struggle is internal and how we individually and collectively as people of faith and values perceive the other, recognize our mutual vulnerability, and act consistently with justice, empathy, and compassion. We need clarity of vision and a sense of purpose to ensure greatly increased efforts to reduce new infections and prevent AIDS-related deaths among the most vulnerable populations at highest risk of HIV acquisition and transmission.

UNAIDS has identified twelve populations that are being left behind by the AIDS response: people living with HIV; adolescent girls and young women; prisoners; migrants; people who inject drugs; sex workers; gay men and other men who have sex with men; transgender people; children and pregnant women living with HIV; displaced persons; people with disabilities; people aged 50 years and older.[11] These communities, which are disproportionately burdened by HIV, are also consistently underserved at every level of service, be it prevention, diagnosis, care, or treatment. We need to acknowledge and address the reality of communities, many of whom face multiple layers of vulnerability in the context of larger structural issues in society, such as racism, homophobia, poverty, and discrimination based on gender and gender identity.

The list is very revealing, as it is diametrically opposite to the powerful and patriarchal sections of society. Where have we chosen to be? Are we following Christ's teaching on the Sermon on the Mount (Matthew 5)? Do we stand with the poor, marginalized, and oppressed or do we "sit in the seat of scoffers" (Ps. 1:1b) and the powerful, and judge?[12]

In what follows, I intentionally lift up three vulnerable communities—adolescent girls and young women; people who inject drugs; and gay men and other men who have sex with men—for discussion. The track record of faith communities in dealing with these communities has been patchy at best, and our willingness to engage communities that are left behind will both determine the success of our struggle against HIV and, I dare say, the very relevance of churches in the future.

Adolescent girls and young women

Are we acknowledging the dignity and the rights of adolescent girls and young women and are we working to prevent their exploitation? More than 5,000 young women and girls acquire HIV every week, the vast majority of them in southern Africa. Adolescent girls and young women in southern Africa acquire HIV five to seven years earlier than their corresponding male peers, and it is evident that age-disparate intergenerational sexual relationships and transactional sex place adolescent girls and young women at extremely high risk of HIV.[13] The 2008 position paper on "Human Rights, HIV/AIDS Prevention, and Gender Equality" by ecumenical development organizations led by the World YWCA states, "To reflect the God given value of each human being, churches should work for an equal and respectful relationship between men and women. To most people of faith religion has a serious influence on their concept of gender roles, human sexuality and marriage. Therefore if FBO's [faith-based organizations] are to participate and contribute to the prevention of further spread of HIV, the issue of gender justice must be taken seriously."[14] Do we strive for "women-led spaces that foster strength through leadership and solidarity towards one vital end: a world where the human rights of women, young women and girls are protected, respected and fulfilled?"[15]

People who inject drugs

Do we recognize that HIV prevalence is 22 times higher among people who inject drugs?[16] UNAIDS estimates that outside sub-Saharan Africa, approximately one third of all HIV infections are related to injecting drug use.[17] Data suggest that an estimated 15.9 million people inject drugs worldwide (2007), with an estimated 3 million of these being HIV-positive.[18]

Fifty years of drug policies aimed at restricting and criminalizing drug use and minor possession have had serious detrimental effects on the health, well-being, and human rights of drug users and the wider public. It is in this context that Prof. Chris Beyer, the current president of the International AIDS Society, with a panel of experts (the authors of the Johns Hopkins-Lancet Commission on Public Health and International Drug Policy), have called for global drug-policy reform. They have provided convincing evidence to show that the "war on drugs" has harmed public health and human rights. They have recommended a move toward a balanced policy, calling on the UN General Assembly to advocate for this. This policy would include:

- Decriminalizing minor, nonviolent drug offenses—use, possession, and petty sale—and strengthen health and social sector alternatives to criminal sanctions.

- Ensuring easy access to harm-reduction services for all who need them as a part of responding to drugs. Opioid substitution therapy (OST), needle substitution programmes (NSP), supervised injection sites, and access to naloxone[19]—brought to a scale adequate to meet demand—should all figure in health services and should include meaningful participation of people who use drugs in planning and implementation.[20]

Gay men and other men who have sex with men

Globally, men who have sex with men (MSM) are 19 times more likely to be living with HIV than the general population.[21] HIV epidemics among MSM are expanding in countries of all incomes, and these epidemics are characterized by high HIV burdens, substantial clustering of infections within networks, and high forces of infection (the force of infection is the rate at which susceptible individuals acquire an infectious disease).[22] Where surveillance has been done, it has shown that men who have sex with men bear a disproportionate burden of HIV. Yet, they continue to be excluded, sometimes systematically, from HIV services because of stigma, discrimination, and criminalization. This situation must change if global control of the HIV epidemic is to be achieved. On both public-health and human-rights grounds, expansion of HIV prevention, treatment, and care to MSM is an urgent imperative.[23]

Although many societies live in denial, alternative sexual orientations beyond heterosexuality are a reality. The results of a scientific study based on a recent survey with nearly 3,000 participating students in southwestern Uganda show that 6 to 8 percent of the men and 10 to 16 percent of the women there have engaged in homosexual relations. Such a prevalence of homosexuality is similar to the situation in most other countries in the world. The surveys also show that homosexual experiences appear to be associated with several health risks, including poor mental health, being the victim of sexual coercion and violence, and engaging in risky sexual behaviour and drug use. People with homosexual experiences also more frequently report their need for, but lack of access to, sexual health counselling. These findings are in the context of widespread strong prejudice against homosexuality in large parts of Ugandan society.[24]

A third of countries around the world (78) still criminalize same-sex conduct, affecting the rights of MSM and other members of the LGBTIQ community. In five countries, homosexuality is punishable by the death penalty. As a result, MSM are less likely to access HIV services for fear of their sexual orientation and identity being revealed.[25]

Can faith communities be quiet or even, at times, part of the society that perpetuates exclusion, oppression, and violence against fellow human beings as a result of homophobia[26] and transphobia?[27] Can we prevent people from living full lives, creating an environment of fear and hatred that forces the affected people to live behind façades, destroying self-esteem and making people susceptible to exploitation and blackmail?

The door of empathy and solidarity with the marginalized and excluded should lead us to action along the path of compassion. Compassion was described in a very deep and touching manner by Henri Nouwen, Donald McNeill, and Douglas Morrison in their 1982 classic *Compassion: A Reflection on the Christian Life*:

> The word *compassion* is derived from the Latin words *pati* and *cum*, which together mean *"suffer with."* Compassion asks us to go where it hurts, to enter into places of pain, to share in brokenness, fear, confusion, and anguish. Compassion requires us to be weak, vulnerable with the vulnerable, powerless with the powerless. Compassion means full immersion in the condition of being human.[28]

The compassionate action should aim for unfettered provision of services focussed on vulnerable communities, ensuring that they can access comprehensive care within an enabling environment that protects individual rights and moves society toward the goal of zero discrimination.

The Danger of HIV Slipping Back into an Exclusive Bio-Medical Realm

With the increasing availability of treatment, there is a tendency not to discuss the situations that make people vulnerable to become infected by HIV. For instance, in Bolivia, where prejudice against homosexuality and transgender persons is widely prevalent, of the 15,000 estimated people living with HIV (given the global trends, perhaps only half of them are aware that they are HIV-positive), only 15 people are open regarding their positive HIV status. Although treatment for HIV is available free of cost, it does not seem to have reduced stigma and discrimination significantly. But readily available treatment allows society sometimes to avoid difficult conversations or facing the reality of the other vulnerabilities experienced by people.[29]

This further underlines the vital role of ensuring that our faith communities provide "safe spaces of grace," so that society can face the realities with dignity and respect. This will be relevant for communities even beyond the age of HIV and AIDS. For AIDS will ultimately be conquered, but human vulnerabilities will remain. Our inability to address them will only make us less prepared as individuals and communities to face new crises.

Connections with other crises

The unique journey with HIV has prepared us to face new challenges. We cannot afford to forget the lessons learned, as humanity will continue to face new and evolving challenges. To that end, I will lift up the linkages and challenges associated with two different epidemics: Ebola and hepatitis C.

The Ebola crisis

The Ebola and HIV epidemics have highlighted the need to strengthen healthcare systems in resource-limited settings. But the systems and networks created and the trainings conducted to combat HIV in West Africa became very valuable in facing the Ebola epidemic. Early in the epidemic, Dr Christoph Benn, director of external relations and the partnerships cluster of the Global Fund, said that the "WCC, churches and ecumenical organizations need to take full responsibility in not only helping to curb the disease but in communicating the right message, in raising awareness and challenging the stigma attached to Ebola."[30] The stigmatization that affected individuals who volunteered in the most courageous way to provide care for Ebola-infected individuals was reminiscent of the stigma that was attached to individuals who worked with HIV or who cared for individuals who were HIV-positive. The lessons learned from the HIV epidemic in terms of community engagement were applied to Ebola. This helped in the implementation of community-awareness sessions and teaching programmes that were necessary to bring about the behavioural and sociocultural changes necessary to override the stigmatization of and discrimination against Ebola-exposed individuals.[31] Faith-based organization (FBOs) moved to respond in the affected countries and prepare in case of outbreaks in other countries, while drawing from their 30 years of experience in HIV interventions.

To respond to the Ebola crisis in West Africa, in September 2014, the WCC, under the leadership of Dr Sue Parry, brought to the table representatives of Christian aid organizations and United Nations agencies to learn from each other and to escalate their efforts to combat the epidemic.[32] The WCC also contributed to the development of the "WHO safe and dignified burial protocol" that was key to reducing Ebola transmission, in partnership with the International Federation of Red Cross and Red Crescent Societies (IFRC) and FBOs, including Islamic Relief, Caritas Internationalis, and World Vision.[33] Coinciding with the 7th biennial conference of the Africa Christian Health Association Platform (ACHAP) in February 2015, WCC and UNAIDS jointly conducted a pre-conference workshop on Ebola and HIV and AIDS in preparedness, response, scale-up, service delivery, and advocacy.[34]

The Ebola crisis has settled down for the time being, but new threats caused by viruses such as Dengue and Zika keep raising their menacing heads, demanding that communities and professionals be ever alert, never forgetting the experiences and capacities developed in battling AIDS.

Overcoming the hepatitis C epidemic

Hepatitis C is a liver disease caused by the hepatitis C virus: the virus can cause both acute and chronic hepatitis infection, ranging in severity from a mild illness lasting a few weeks to a serious, lifelong illness. An estimated 130 to 150 million people globally have chronic hepatitis C infection. A significant number of those who are chronically infected will develop liver cirrhosis or liver cancer. Approximately 500,000 people die each year from hepatitis C-related liver diseases.[35] The hepatitis C virus is a blood-borne virus and the most common modes of infection are through unsafe injection practices; inadequate sterilization of medical equipment; and the transfusion of unscreened blood and blood products. Transmission rarely occurs from exposure to other infected body fluids, such as semen, unless diseases such as HIV compromise one's immunity. Antiviral medicines can cure approximately 90 percent of persons with hepatitis C infection, thereby reducing the risk of death from liver cancer and cirrhosis, but access to diagnosis and treatment is low. There is currently no vaccine for hepatitis C; however, research in this area is ongoing.

HIV and hepatitis C virus (HCV) transmission networks are closely linked. Evidence shows that the transmission networks of HIV and HCV are correlated and overlap even beyond the degree that can be expected by demographic variables such as risk group, geography, sex, and age.[36]

When the U.S. Food and Drug Administration (FDA) approved the revolutionary new hepatitis C virus (HCV) treatment sofosbuvir, in December 2013, it immediately sparked global headlines and controversy. The treatment, part of a class of drugs known as direct-acting antivirals (DAAs), was associated with cure rates of over 90 percent in clinical trials, nearly double the rate of previous treatments. However, sofosbuvir's initial price tag of US $1,000 a pill, or US $84,000 for a 12-week course of treatment, put it far beyond the reach of nearly all of the approximately 160 million people chronically infected with HCV globally—including approximately 5 million people living with HIV who are affected by HCV. With the strong experience of successful advocacy to bring down the cost of HIV medication worldwide, advocates began campaigning to bring prices down and facilitate greater treatment access. In September 2014, Gilead, the manufacturer of sofosbuvir, signed a voluntary license agreement allowing seven (and later eleven) Indian generic companies to sell a less expensive generic version of sofosbuvir in 91 lower-income countries, a number that was expanded to 101 in August 2015. However, this list excludes many of the world's hardest-hit middle-income countries, such as China. And even in the included countries, a course of treatment would cost at least US $900, which is still far above what many low-income countries can afford on a large scale. It is also much higher than the estimated US $120 that British researchers have concluded it could cost to manufacture a 12-week course of therapy. While the introduction of sofosbuvir by generic Indian companies has been a positive development, access to the medicine still remains a key challenge in many countries, and advocates are working hard to improve that access.[37]

Dr Gareth Owen calls hepatitis C infection the new elephant in the room, with significant experiences of stigma and discrimination experienced by those affected.[38] Apart from advocacy to bring down the price of medication, the experiences from the work on HIV and AIDS will also help us to organize communities of people living with chronic hepatitis C infection and to work toward curing them and to work against stigma and discrimination.

Conclusion

In conclusion, as we look to the future, we need to continue to analyze critically the needs of society to end AIDS and follow a three-pronged approach for our onward journey:

1. Hold our governments, our faith communities, public and private institutions, corporations, the international communities, and ourselves accountable to the commitments made to overcome HIV in order to close the gap between policies and action. We should continue to work against stigma and discrimination and advocate for the allocation of adequate resources for holistic and comprehensive HIV response in every country, ensuring unhindered access to all communities.

2. Ensure that our faith communities are "safe spaces of grace"; facilitate society's addressing human vulnerabilities that make us to susceptible to HIV and many existing and potential future challenges; and work to ensure that churches remain preferentially committed to the poor and the marginalized.

3. Implement the rights- and dignity-based and inclusive approach we have used successfully to control HIV in existing and other potential future challenges.

May the memory of over 30 million people who have lost their lives to AIDS and AIDS-related illnesses remind us of the high cost humanity has paid for this painful and costly journey!

May we never forget!

May the lives of the 37 million people living with HIV inspire us to continue this ecumenical journey with compassion and competence!

May we always respond in a timely and adequate manner!

May we as individuals and communities who continue to be vulnerable to HIV and many forms of suffering and injustice commit ourselves to look to the future with hope and strive for a better tomorrow, with courage!

May the reign of God be established here and now!

Historical Timeline

1981[1]

- On June 5, the CDC's Morbidity and Mortality Weekly Report publishes the first mention of what later is determined to be HIV. The report mentions five cases of pneumocystis carinii pneumonia in young men.

- By the end of the year, there are 270 reported cases of severe immune deficiency among gay men—121 of whom have died.

- Six men in New York set up a hotline, receiving 100 calls the first night. The hotline becomes the world's first HIV and AIDS service organization, the Gay Men's Health Crisis.

1982

- Introduction of the term "acquired immunodeficiency syndrome," or AIDS.

- Disease reported in hemophiliacs and Haitians, leading many to believe it originated in Haiti.

- Doctors in Uganda report cases of a new, fatal wasting disease locally known as "slim."[2]

1983

- AIDS reported among the female partners of males with the disease, suggesting it could be passed on via heterosexual sex.

- Doctors at the Pasteur Institute in France report the discovery of a new retrovirus called Lymphadenopathy-Associated Virus (or LAV) that could be the cause of AIDS.[3]

- The WHO holds its first meeting to assess the global AIDS situation and begin international surveillance.

- The WHO asks the WCC, in the context of their ongoing, official relationship since 1975, to raise awareness among the churches regarding the emerging disease called AIDS.

1984

- The U.S. National Cancer Institute announces they have found the cause of AIDS, the retrovirus HTLV-III. In a joint conference with the Pasteur Institute, they announce that LAV and HTLV-III are identical and the likely cause of AIDS.

- The first conference of the WCC on AIDS is held in Geneva in June.

1985

- The U.S. Food and Drug Administration (FDA) approves and licenses the first commercial blood test, ELISA, to detect antibodies to the virus.

- Actor Rock Hudson announces that he is dying of AIDS.

- The U.S. HHS and the WHO host the first (I) International AIDS Conference in Atlanta, Georgia.

1986

- The WCC's Executive Committee meeting in Reykjavik, Iceland, 15–19 September 1986, makes prophetic recommendations to churches to face up to AIDS with the clarity of vision and in truth.

- II International AIDS Conference—Paris

1987

- The WCC publishes and distributes the two popular key resources authored by Dr Birgitta Rubenson: *What Is AIDS? A Manual for Health Workers*, and *Learning about HIV and AIDS: A Manual for Pastors and Teachers*.

- The conference "Theological and Ethical Issues Related to AIDS," is held in Toronto, Canada, 23–25 October 1987, co-sponsored by The Canadian Council of Churches, The National Council of Churches of Christ in the U.S.A., and the WCC.

- The FDA approves AZT, the first antiretroviral drug for treating AIDS.

- Activist Larry Kramer creates the AIDS Coalition to Unleash Power (ACT UP). ACT UP leads many nonviolent protests through the 1990s.

- Activist Cleve Jones makes the first panel for the AIDS Memorial Quilt. To date, the quilt contains more than 48,000 panels.

- III International AIDS Conference—Washington, D.C.

1988

- IV International AIDS Conference—Stockholm, Sweden. This conference marks the end of the period when the main focus was on biomedical aspects of HIV and AIDS. The "Face of AIDS" is introduced at the conference as a forum of people living with HIV, patients, and civil society now being included in the debate.

1989

- V International AIDS Conference—Montreal, Canada. Theme: "The Scientific and Social Challenge of AIDS." Activists occupy centre stage during the conference: Canadians activists protest the lack of a federally funded AIDS strategy; U.S. activists denounce the U.S. entry ban for people living with HIV, and both want a greater involvement in the conference. During the same conference, Zambian president Kenneth Kaunda reveals that his son died of AIDS in 1986, becoming the first African leader to speak about AIDS in his own family.

1990

- The WCC publishes *A Guide to HIV/AIDS Pastoral Counselling*, edited by Rev. Jorge Maldonado, with support from the AIDS Working Group guided by Dr. Elinda Senturias.

- VI International AIDS Conference—San Francisco, USA. Theme: "AIDS in the Nineties: From Science to Policy." The conference sees huge protests due to the weak U.S. federal government response to the epidemic and a lack of effective treatment for people living with HIV.

1991

- Singer Paul Jabara starts the Red Ribbon Foundation, which begins distributing ribbons as a symbol of tolerance for those living with HIV and AIDS.

- Magic Johnson, three-time National Basketball Association (NBA) most valuable player, announces that he has HIV and will retire from the Los Angeles Lakers.

- VII International AIDS Conference—Florence, Italy. Theme: "Science Challenging AIDS." Experts from Africa and India discuss the growing burden of the epidemic in their regions.

1992

- VIII International AIDS Conference—Amsterdam, Netherlands. Theme: "A World United Against AIDS."

1993

- The critically acclaimed movie *Philadelphia*, starring Tom Hanks and Denzel Washington, is released. In the drama, a man with AIDS (Hanks) is fired by a conservative law firm because of his condition, so he hires a homophobic lawyer (Washington) to sue.

- IX International AIDS Conference—Berlin. This meeting highlights the walls between HIV-positive and HIV-negative people and between rich and poor.

- Disappointing year in HIV research: the results of the Concorde trial of AZT monotherapy shows no medium- or long-term benefit. Also, the economic impact of AIDS epidemic is becoming increasingly obvious.

1994

- The WCC Central Committee meeting in Johannesburg, South Africa, mandates the formation of a consultative group to conduct a study on HIV and AIDS. Consultative group on HIV and AIDS is formed and headed by Dr Christoph Benn (then working for DIFÄM)

- Elizabeth Glaser, wife of actor Paul Michael Glaser, loses her battle with AIDS, and her Pediatric AIDS Foundation is renamed. Glaser started the children's research foundation after she contracted HIV while giving birth.

- X International AIDS Conference—Yokohama, Japan. Theme: "The Global Challenge of AIDS: Together for the Future." Future conferences are held on a biannual basis.

1995

- To correspond with the fourth World Conference on Women, Beijing, China, the WCC draws together the experiences of women, health, and the challenge of HIV from Brazil, Argentina, Costa Rica, Chile, India, Thailand, Papua New Guinea, Uganda, DRC (Zaire), Tanzania, and the USA. Because China had a travel ban on people living with HIV, the WCC conducts the meeting in India.

- The WCC publishes *Contact*, no. 144, "Women and AIDS: Building Healing Communities."

1996

- The landmark result of the WCC consultative group's global study on AIDS is reported to the WCC Central Committee. which adopts a statement based on the report.

- The Joint United Nations Programme on AIDS (UNAIDS) is established by the United Nations. It combines experts from six agencies to fight the AIDS epidemic.

- The WCC publishes *Love in a Time of AIDS: Women, Health and the Challenge of HIV*, by Gillian Paterson

- XI International AIDS Conference—Vancouver, Canada. Theme: "One World, One Hope." Significant treatment breakthrough: highly active anti-retroviral therapy (HAART) sees mortality and morbidity among patients drop dramatically and the prognosis for HIV disease shift from almost certain fatality to a chronic illness. The term "Lazarus syndrome" is used to describe patients who return from the brink of death to good health. After the excitement, though, it becomes quickly evident that while the therapy can be used widely in high-income countries, in the areas of the world where the epidemic is more devastating, the access to it is very limited.

- The Contextual Bible Study of Tamar's rape, as given by 2 Samuel 13:12-18, is developed by the Ujamaa Centre for Biblical and Theological Community Development and Research, based at the University of Kwazulu-Natal, Pietermaritzburg

1997

- The WCC publishes the results of their consultative group's global study on AIDS, *Facing AIDS: The Challenge, the Churches' Response*, in English, French and Spanish. An accompanying study guide, *Facing AIDS: Education in the Context of Vulnerability*, by Karen Anderson (EPES) and Gert Rüppell (WCC), is also published in the three languages.

- The WCC co-publishes *Confronting AIDS Together: Participatory methods in addressing the HIV/AIDS epidemic: including learning from the WCC experience in East and Central Africa*, by Anne Skjelmerud and Christopher Tusubira.

- In the USA, antiretroviral drugs like Truvada have helped control the AIDS epidemic and the U.S. death rate from the disease declines.

1998

- 8th WCC General Assembly, Harare, Zimbabwe, focuses on the theme "Turn to God—Rejoice in Hope." Churches in Africa call for solidarity in the face of HIV.

- XII International AIDS Conference—Geneva, Switzerland. Theme: "Bridging the Gap." This meeting addresses the gaps in treatment between the wealthy and the poor, gaps in power and autonomy between men and women, and the gap between governmental authorities and civil society.

1999

- The WHO announced that HIV and AIDS was the fourth biggest cause of death worldwide and the number one killer in Africa, with an estimated 33 million people living with HIV and 14 million people who have died from AIDS since the start of the epidemic.

2000

- The WCC along with its ecumenical partners initiate the Ecumenical Advocacy Alliance (EAA) as an international network of churches and church-related organizations committed to campaigning together on common concerns. HIV and AIDS is chosen as one of the two pressing issues around which to do global advocacy. HIV remains one of the EAA's two campaigns to date.

- XIII International AIDS Conference—Durban, South Africa. Theme: "Breaking the Silence."
  - The focus is placed on the staggering impact of the epidemic in sub-Saharan Africa and on the inequity in treatment access between the developed and the developing world.

  - South African President Thabo Mbeki declares he doubts AIDS occurred in South Africa. The minister of health shares the same ideas and forbids the use of antiretrovirals to prevent mother-to-child transmission.

  - These declarations prompt 5,000 scientists from around the world to publish the "Durban Declaration," confirming the overwhelming scientific evidence about the etiology of AIDS.

- The Durban conference proves to be a unique opportunity to address both treatment inequity and denialism.

- During the closing ceremony, Nelson Mandela speaks against the irresponsibility of the South African government on AIDS.

2001

- UN General Assembly Special Session on HIV/AIDS (UNGASS 2001) results in a Declaration of Commitment, which establishes ambitious goals for treatment, prevention, and care.

- UNAIDS marks the 20th anniversary of the first report on HIV. Executive director Peter Piot says, "in just 20 years AIDS has infected 60 million people, killed 22 million and achieved the status of the most devastating epidemic in human history."

- WCC conducts several regional consultations on HIV and AIDS, with church leaders and ecumenical partners, including
  - in East Africa, in Mukono, Kampala, Uganda, 15–17 January, in collaboration with All Africa Conference of Churches;
  - in Southern Africa, in Johannesburg, South Africa, 26–29 March, in collaboration with South African Council of Churches;
  - in West Africa, in Dakar, Senegal, 23–25 April, in collaboration with All Africa Conference of Churches and Medical Assistance Programme (MAP International).

- This series concludes with the "Global Consultation on the Ecumenical Response to the Challenge of HIV/AIDS," in Africa, Nairobi, Kenya, 25–28 November, which produces a "Plan of Action," giving rise to WCC-EHAIA in 2002.

- After generic-drug manufacturers offer to produce discounted, generic forms of HIV and AIDS drugs for developing countries, several major pharmaceutical manufacturers agree to further reduce drug prices. The World Trade Organization (WTO) announces,the Doha Declaration, which allows developing countries to manufacture generic medications to combat public-health crises like HIV and AIDS.

2002

- The WCC launches the Ecumenical HIV and AIDS Initiative in Africa (EHAIA).
- Founding of the African Network of Religious Leaders Living With and/or Personally Affected by HIV and AIDS (ANERELA+).
- First rapid HIV test, which produces results in less than 20 minutes.
- The Global Fund approves its first round of grants, totalling $600 million.
- Combinations of events at the turn of the millennium, including international commitment and political will, intense activism, and corporate philanthropy in the pharmaceutical sector, lead to dramatic reductions in the price of antiretrovirals.
- XIV International AIDS Conference—Barcelona, Spain. Theme: "Knowledge and Commitment for Action"

2003

- First of a new type of anti-HIV drug—enfuvirtide (Fuzeon)—designed to prevent the entry of HIV into human cells, approved by the FDA.
- Bill and Melinda Gates Foundation awards a $60 million grant to the International Partnership for Microbicides to support research and development of microbicides to prevent transmission of HIV.
- WHO announces the "3 by 5" initiative, to bring treatment to 3 million people by 2005.

2004

- U.S. president George W. Bush launches PEPFAR, the U.S. President's Emergency Plan to combat AIDS worldwide.
- The WHO launches "Guidance on Ethics and Equitable Access to HIV Treatment and Care."
- An estimated 700,000 people receive antiretroviral drugs in developing countries.

- XV International AIDS Conference—Bangkok, Thailand. Theme: "Access for All."

- The first Interfaith Ecumenical Pre-Conference is organized by EAA, with active engagement of faith-based organiztions during the International AIDS Conference.

2005

- For the first time, the FDA approves a generic AIDS drug made by a foreign country, allowing PEPFAR to provide cheaper medications in Africa and developing countries around the world.

- The patent on AZT also reaches an end, allowing more generic versions of the drug.

- Joint ILO (International Labor Organization)/WHO guidelines on health services and HIV and AIDS.

- Policy and programming guide for HIV and AIDS prevention and care among injecting drug users,

- The Conference on World Mission and Evangelism (CWME) —Athens. Theme: "Come, Holy Spirit, Heal and Reconcile."

2006

- 9th WCC General Assembly, Porto Alegre, Brazil. Theme: "God in Your Grace, Transform the World."

- The WCC issues a statement, "Churches' Compassionate Response to HIV and AIDS."

- Establishment of the International Network of Religious Leaders—lay and ordained, women and men—Living with, or Personally Affected, by HIV (INERELA+).

- The United Nations convenes a follow-up meeting and issues a progress report on the implementation of the Declaration of Commitment on HIV/AIDS Exit Disclaimer.

- Singer Bono, of the rock group U2, launches Product Red. Profits from the line of consumer goods are designated to fight the AIDS epidemic worldwide.

- Bill Gates announces that he will step down as the head of Microsoft to donate his time to the Gates Foundation, the largest private source of funding in the fight against HIV and AIDS.

- The FDA approves Atripla, the first effective one-a-day pill to treat HIV.

- Male circumcision is found to reduce the risk of female-to-male HIV transmission by 60 percent. Since then, the WHO and UNAIDS have emphasised that male circumcision should be considered in areas with high HIV and low male circumcision prevalence.

- XVI International AIDS Conference—Toronto, Canada. Theme: "A Time To Deliver"

2007

- Establishment of the Africa Christian Health Association Platform (ACHAP).
- Guidelines provided by the WHO on:
  - Global scale-up of the prevention of mother-to-child transmission of HIV;
  - Provider-initiated HIV testing and counselling in health facilities;
  - Post-exposure prophylaxis to prevent HIV infection.

2008

- XVII International AIDS Conference, Mexico City, Mexico. Theme: "Universal Action Now."

- Panama repeals law criminalizing homosexuality, the last Latin American country to do so.

- China lifts its ban on people with HIV travelling to the country.

2010

- XVII International AIDS Conference—Vienna, Austria. Theme: "Rights Here, Right Now."

- The first positive demonstration that topical antiretrovirals can prevent HIV (CAPRISA 004).

- "Framework for Dialogue" emerges from the summit of High-Level Religious Leaders held in the Netherlands—the successful format of a dialogue between religious leaders and people living with HIV at the national level. Partners include EAA, GNPINERELA+, and UNAIDS.

- A third phase of a PrEP (pre-exposure prophylaxis) trial reveals that drugs used to treat HIV may also be effective in preventing infection. Subjects taking a once-daily antiretroviral pill are shown to be 44 percent less likely to contract HIV after male-to-male sex.

- The Ecumenical Pharmaceutical Network (EPN) publishes *HIV and AIDS Treatment Literacy Guide for Church Leaders*.

- U.S. government officially lifts its HIV travel and immigration ban.

2011

- Results from the HPTN 052 trial shows that early initiation of antiretroviral treatment reduces the risk of HIV transmission by 96 percent among serodiscordant heterosexual couples (i.e., one partner being uninfected).

- FDA approves Complera, the second all-in-one fixed-dose combination tablet, expanding the treatment options available for people living with HIV.

2012

- XIX International AIDS Conference—Washington, DC. Theme: "Turning the Tide Together." A main focus is the launch of "Towards an HIV Cure."

- UNAIDS announces that new HIV infections have dropped more than 50 percent in 25 low- and middle-income countries, and the number of people getting antiretroviral treatment has increased 63 percent in the past two years. More than 34 million people are still living with HIV.

- Researchers announce they have "functionally cured" a Mississippi toddler of HIV. They believe that early intervention—in this case within 30 hours of birth—with three antiviral drugs is key to the outcome.

- The WHO recommends antiretroviral treatment as prevention (TASP) of HIV and TB.

- For the first time, the majority of people eligible for treatment are receiving it (54%).

2013

- UNAIDS reports that AIDS-related deaths have fallen 30 percent since their peak in 2005.

- An estimated 35 million people are living with HIV.

- 10th WCC Assembly, Busan, the Republic of Korea. Theme: "God of Life, Lead Us to Justice and Peace."

- During the assembly, "safe space" is created for dialogue on human sexuality, featuring stories of pain, exclusion, and violence faced by sexual minorities in many parts of the world.

2014

- The WHO issues "Guidelines on HIV/STI Prevention and Treatment" for men who have sex with men, sex workers, and people who use drugs, and the 2014 "Consolidated Guidelines on HIV Prevention, Diagnosis, Care, and Treatment for Key Populations."

- UNAIDS "Fast Track" targets call for the dramatic scaling-up of HIV prevention and treatment programmes to avert 28 million new infections and end the epidemic as a public-health issue by 2030.

- UNAIDS launches the ambitious 90-90-90 targets, which aim for 90 percent of people living with HIV to be diagnosed, 90 percent to be accessing antiretroviral treatment, and 90 percent to achieve viral suppression by 2020.

- XX International AIDS Conference—Melbourne, Australia. Theme: "Stepping Up the Pace."

2015

- UNAIDS announces that the Millennium Development Goal (MDG) relating to HIV and AIDS has been reached six months ahead of schedule. The target of MDG 6—halting and reversing the spread of HIV—saw 15 million people receive treatment.

- The WHO launches new treatment guidelines recommending that all people living with HIV should receive antiretroviral treatment, regardless of their CD4 count, and as soon as possible after their diagnosis.

- UNAIDS releases their 2016–2021 strategy in line with the new Sustainable Development Goals (SDGs), which call for an acceleration in the global HIV response to reach critical HIV prevention and treatment targets and achieve zero discrimination.

Abbreviations

AACC	All Africa Conference of Churches
ACHAP	African Christian Health Association Platform
ACT UP	AIDS Coalition to Unleash Power
AIDS	Acquired Immunodeficiency Syndrome
AINA	Asian Interfaith Network on AIDS
ANERELA+	African Network of Religious Leaders Living With and/ or Personally Affected by HIV and AIDS
ANERTHA	African Network of Higher Education and Research in Religion, Theology, HIV and AIDS
ARHAP	African Religious Health Assets Program
ART	Antiretroviral Therapy
ARV	Antiretrovirals
AZT	Zidovudine
CABSA	Christian AIDS Bureau of Southern Africa
CBS	Contextual Bible Study
CCA	Christian Conference of Asia
CCIA	Commission of the Churches on International Affairs
CDC	U.S. Centers for Disease Control and Prevention
CHA	Christian Health Association (or Organization)
CHART	Collaborative for HIV and AIDS, Religion and Theology
CLAI	Latin American Council of Churches

CMC	WCC's Christian Medical Commission
CWME	Commission on World Mission and Evangelism
DAA	Direct-acting antiviral
DIFÄM	Deutsches Institut für Ärztliche Mission (German Institute for Medical Mission)
EHAIA	Ecumenical HIV and AIDS Initiatives and Advocacy
EKD	Evangelical Church in Germany (Evangelische Kirche in Deutschland)
EPES	Evangelical Lutheran Church of Chile's Program for Health Education
EPN	Ecumenical Pharmaceutical Network
FBO	Faith-based organization
FDA	U.S. Food and Drug Administration
FGM	Female genital mutilation
FHI 360	Family Health International 360
FOCAGIFO	Friends of Canon Gideon Foundation
FOCCISA	Cooperation of the Fellowship of Council of Churches in Southern Africa
GNP+	Global Network of People Living with HIV
HCV	Hepatitis C Virus
HCT	HIV and AIDS Counselling and Testing
HHS	U.S. Department of Health and Human Services
HIV	Human Immunodeficiency Virus
HLM	High-Level Meeting
ICAAP	International Congress on AIDS in Asia and the Pacific
IEC	Information, Education and Communication
IFRC	International Federation of Red Cross and Red Crescent Societies
IICA	Indian Interfaith Coalition on AIDS
ILO	International Labor Organization
INERELA+	International Network of Religious Leaders Living with or Personally Affected by HIV or AIDS
INHAT	Interfaith Network on HIV and AIDS in Thailand
INTERNA	Indonesian Interfaith Network on AIDS

ISER	Institute for Religious Studies
LAV	Lymphadenopathy-Associated Virus
LGBTIQ	Lesbian/gay/bisexual/transgender/intersexed/queer
LWF	Lutheran World Federation
MAP International	Medical Assistance Programme International
MDG	Millennium Development Goal
MINA	Myanmar Interfaith Network on HIV and AIDS
MSM	Men who have sex with men
NEK	North Elbian Evangelical Lutheran Church (Nordelbische Evangelisch-Lutherische Kirche
NGO	Nongovernmental organizations
NORAD	Norwegian Agency for Development Cooperation
NSP	Needle Substitution Programmes
PEPFAR	President's Emergency Plan for AIDS Relief
PLWHA	People Living with HIV and AIDS
PWID	People who inject drugs
PMCT/PMTCT	Prevention of Mother-to-Child Transmission
OVC	Orphans and Vulnerable Children
OST	Opioid Substitution Therapy
PrEP	Pre-exposure prophylaxis
SDG	Sustainable Development Goal
SGBV	Sexual and gender-based violence
SPSARV	Special Program on Substance Abuse and Related Violence (UMC)
SRHR	Sexual and Reproductive Health and Rights
STI	Sexually transmitted infection
SWIM	Sex Workers in Myanmar
TASP	Treatment as prevention
TB	Tuberculosis
TWG	Technical working group
UEM	United Evangelical Mission
UMC	United Methodist Church
UNAIDS	Joint United Nations Programme on HIV and AIDS

UNDP	United Nations Development Programme
UNFPA	United Nations Population Fund
UNGASS	UN General Assembly Special Session
UNICEF	United Nations Children's Fund
USAID	United States Agency for International Development
VAW/g	Violence against women and girls
VCT	Voluntary Counselling and Testing
WCC	World Council of Churches
WCC-EAA	WCC-Ecumenical Advocacy Alliance
WHO	World Health Organization
WTO	World Trade Organization
YWCA	Young Women's Christian Association

Notes

Preface

1. "Fast Track to Ending AIDS," 2016 High-Level Meeting on Ending Aids, United Nations General Assembly, New York, 8–10 June 2016, http://www.unaids.org/sites/default/files/media_asset/2016HighLevelMeeting_en.pdf.

2. AIDS.gov, "How Do You Get HIV or AIDS?" 31 December 2015, https://www.aids.gov/hiv-aids-basics/hiv-aids-101/how-you-get-hiv-aids/.

3. WHO, "Effectiveness of Sterile Needle and Syringe Programming in Reducing HIV/AIDS among Injecting Drug Users," Evidence for Action Technical Papers (Geneva: World Health Organization, 2004), http://www.who.int/hiv/pub/prev_care/effectivenesssterileneedle.pdf.

4. "Achievements: The WCC and the Ecumenical Movement," https://www.oikoumene.org/en/about-us/achievements.

Chapter 1: Connectedness and Accountability

1. Interview with George Lemopoulos, Deputy General Secretary, WCC, 2 February 2016.

2. Calle Almedal, "A Thirty-Year Personal Journey with HIV," *The Ecumenical Review* 63, no. 4 (December 2011): 369–77.

3. CMC (Christian Medical Commission), "The Beginnings—Tübingen 1, 1964," (Geneva: World Council of Churches, 1979).

4. J. C. McGilvray, *The Quest for Health and Wholeness* (Tübingen: German Institute for Medical Missions, 1981).

5. WCC/CMC, "Introduction to the Microfilm Collection," http://web.library.yale.edu/sites/default/files/files/WCCChristianMedicalCommission.pdf.

6. WHO, "Report of International Conference on Primary Health Care, Alma-Ata, USSR" (Geneva: WHO Publications, 1978); idem, "The World Health Report 2002: Reducing Risks, Promoting Healthy Life" (Geneva: WHO Publications, 2002), http://www.who.int/whr/2002/en/.

7. Socrates Litsios, "The Christian Medical Commission and the Development of WHO's Primary Health Care Approach," *American Journal of Public Health* 94, no. 11 (November 2004): 1884–93, http://www.ncbi.nlm.nih.gov/pmc/articles/PMC1448555/.

8. Center for Disease Control, "Current Trends Prevention of Acquired Immune Deficiency Syndrome (AIDS): Report of Inter-Agency Recommendations," *Morbidity and Mortality Weekly Report* (MMWR) 32, no. 8 (4 March 1983): 101–103, http://www.cdc.gov/mmwr/preview/mmwrhtml/00001257.htm.

9. Dr. Fakhry Assaad, until his death on 28 December 1986, was the director, division of communicable diseases, WHO, Geneva.

10. Dickens Warfield, "Missionary Impossible: The Life and Work of Cecile De Sweemer" (2006), http://www.butoke.org/MissionaryImpossible.pdf.

11. At the consultation on "Theological and Ethical Issues Related to AIDS," in Toronto, Canada, 23–25 October 1987, co-sponsored by the Canadian Council of Churches, the National Council of Churches of Christ in the U.S.A, and the WCC.

12. Dr Jonathan Max Mann (1947–1998) founded the WHO's Global Programme for AIDS in 1986 and headed the department until his departure from WHO in 1990. Dr. Mann was a pioneer in his advocacy for combining public health, ethics, and human rights.

13. Cecile De Sweemer, "AIDS: The Global Crisis," in David G. Hallman, ed., *AIDS Issues: Confronting the Challenge* (New York: Pilgrim Press, 1989), 50.

14. Susan E. Davies, "Oppression and Resurrection Faith," in Letty R. Russell, ed., *The Church with AIDS: Renewal in the Midst of Crisis* (Louisville: Westminster John Knox, 1990), 90.

15. Anne Skjelmerud and Christopher Tusubira, *Confronting AIDS Together: Participatory methods in addressing the HIV/AIDS epidemic: including learning from the WCC experience in East and Central Africa* (Oslo/Geneva: Centre for Partnership Development, in collaboration with WCC, 1997).

16. De Sweemer, "AIDS: The Global Crisis," 31–32.

17. Gillian Paterson, *Love in a Time of AIDS: Women, Health and the Challenge of HIV*, Risk Books (Geneva: WCC Publications, 1996); also published in the USA under the title *Women in the Time of AIDS* (Maryknoll, NY: Orbis, 1997).

18. "Women and AIDS: Building Healing Communities," *Contact* 144 (August-September 1995), http://www.oikoumene.org/en/what-we-do/health-and-healing/144AugSept1995WomenandAIDSbuildinghealingcommunities.pdf.

19. Christoph Benn, "The Impact of CMC on Health Care in Industrialised Countries," in WCC, *The Vision and the Future of CMC: 25 Years of CMC* (Geneva: CMC—Churches Action for Health/WCC Publications, 1995).

20. WCC, *Facing AIDS: The Challenge, the Churches' Response*, a WCC Study Document (Geneva: WCC Publications, 1997; reprinted in 2000, 2001, 2002 and 2004).

21. Karen Anderson and Gert Rüppell, *Facing AIDS: Education in the Context of Vulnerability HIV/AIDS* (Geneva: WCC Publications, 1999), http://

hivhealthclearinghouse.unesco.org/sites/default/files/resources/bie_world_council_churches_facing_aids_en.pdf.

22. UNAIDS/WHO, "A History of the HIV/AIDS Epidemic with Emphasis on Africa," 5 September 2003, http://www.un.org/esa/population/publications/adultmort/UNAIDS_WHOPaper2.pdf.

23. De Sweemer, "AIDS: The Global Crisis," 33.

24. UNAIDS/WHO, "AIDS Epidemic Update: December 1998," UNAIDS Joint United Nations Programme on HIV/AIDS, http://data.unaids.org/Publications/IRC-pub06/epiupdate98_en.pdf.

25. Alexander Rödlach, "Home-Based Care for People Living with AIDS in Zimbabwe: Voluntary Caregivers' Motivations and Concerns," *African Journal of AIDS Research* 8, no. 4 (2009): 423–31.

26. WCC, "HIV and AIDS Curriculum for Theological Institutions in Africa," 2002, https://www.oikoumene.org/en/folder/documents-pdf/curriculum-for-theological-institutions-eng.pdf.

27. WCC, *Facing AIDS: Education in the Context of Vulnerability* (see n. 21 above).

28. Mindy J. Roseman and Sofia Gruskin, "The UNGASS Declaration of Commitment: One Year Later," *Canadian HIV/AIDS Policy and Law Review* 8, no. 1 (April 2003).

29. Plenary presentation at the United Nations General Assembly Special Session on HIV/AIDS by Dr. Christoph Benn, representing the Commission of the Churches on International Affairs of the World Council of Churches, 27 June 2001.

30. UNAIDS, "A Report of a Theological Workshop Focusing on HIV- and AIDS-related Stigma, 8th to 11th December 2003, Windhoek, Namibia, February 2005," http://data.unaids.org/Publications/IRC-pub06/jc1056_theological-report_en.pdf.

31. "The Nadi Declaration," A Statement of the World Council of Churches' Pacific Member Churches on HIV/AIDS, 2004, https://www.oikoumene.org/en/folder/documents-pdf/nadideclaration2006.pdf.

32. WCC, "The Church and HIV/AIDS in Latin America and the Caribbean," 1 February 2004, https://www.oikoumene.org/en/resources/documents/other-ecumenical-bodies/church-statements-on-hivaids/latin-american-regional-meeting.

33. WCC, "Message from Latin American Churches, Church Organisations and Programmes on World AIDS Day 2004," 1 December 2004, https://www.oikoumene.org/en/resources/documents/other-ecumenical-bodies/church-statements-on-hivaids/latin-american-churches-and-organizations.

34. Caribbean Conference of Churches, "Guidelines for Caribbean Faith-Based Organisations on Developing Policies and Action Plans to Deal with HIV/AIDS," http://www.ccc-caribe.org/eng/resources.htm.

35. WCC, "Report on Public Issues: Statement on Churches' Compassionate Response to HIV and AIDS," 6 September 2006, http://www.oikoumene.org/en/resources/documents/central-committee/2006/report-on-public-issues.

36. Anglican Communion across Africa, "Our Vision, Our Hope: The First Step," 22 August 2002, https://www.oikoumene.org/en/resources/documents/other-ecumenical-bodies/church-statements-on-hivaids/anglican-communion-africa.

37. "Pastoral Letter from the Primates of the Anglican Communion," Anglican Communion News Service, 27 May 2003, http://www.anglicannews.org/news/2003/05/pastoral-letter-from-the-primates-of-the-anglican-communion.aspx.

38. In 2012 the NEK, the Evangelical Lutheran Church of Mecklenburg, and the Pomeranian Evangelical Church merged to becomes the Evangelical Lutheran Church in Northern Germany.

39. Evangelical Church in Germany, "For a Life with Dignity: The Global Threat of HIV/AIDS: Possible Courses of Action for the Church," A Study by the Evangelical Church in Germany's Advisory Commission on Sustainable Development, EKD Texts 91, Hanover, 2007, https://www.ekd.de/english/download/aids_text_91.pdf.

40. Sonja Weinreich and Christoph Benn, *AIDS—Meeting the Challenge: Data, Facts, Background* (Geneva: WCC Publications, 2004); trans. of *AIDS: Eine Krankheit verändert die Welt. Daten–Fakten–Hintergründe* (Frankfurt am Main: Verlag Otto Lembeck, 2003).

41. Olav Fykse Tveit, presentation at "Religious Leadership in Response to HIV: A Summit of High Level Religious Leaders," 22–23 March 2010, Amsterdam, http://www.e-alliance.ch/en/l/hivaids/summit-of-high-level-religious/summit-documents/index.html.

Chapter 2: Back to Basics

1. Manoj Kurian, "Healing," in Kenneth R Ross, Jooseop Keum, Kyriaki Avtzi, and Roderick Hewitt, eds., *Ecumenical Missiology: Changing Landscapes and New Conceptions of Mission*, Regnum Edinburgh Centenary Series (Oxford: Regnum Press, 2016).

2. "The Healing Mission of the Church," Preparatory Paper no. 11, in Jacques Matthey, ed., *Come Holy Spirit, Heal and Reconcile! Called in Christ to Be Reconciling and Healing Communities*, Report of the WCC Conference on World Mission and Evangelism, Athens, Greece, 9–16 May 2005 (Geneva: WCC Publications, 2008), 91–112, at 103.

3. Rebecca J. Welch Kline and Nelya J. McKenzie, "HIV/AIDS, Women, and Threads of Discrimination: A Tapestry of Disenfranchisement," in Eileen Berlin Ray, ed., *Communication and Disenfranchisement: Social Health Issues and Implications* (Mahwah, NJ: Routledge, 1996), 365–86.

4. Quoted from the "Plan of Action" formulated at the "Global Consultation on Ecumenical Responses to the Challenges of HIV/AIDS in Africa," Nairobi, Kenya, 25–28 November 2001.

5. For years, I could not reconcile myself with the teaching "Blessed are those who mourn, for they will be comforted" (Matt. 5:4). Are we supposed to be mourning all the time? Or is it just a blessing for those who are facing tough times? It became clearer after I conducted a personal research project on "Encounters with God" (2005–2006). I

interviewed 100 individuals from all over the world on their experiences and interpretation of "being in the presence of God." Seventy-five percent of the persons I interviewed reported experiencing the presence of God during intensely challenging times. At any given time, there is enough suffering that is going on in the world. To be empathetic and to step outside our own comfort zone, in solidarity with those who are suffering, seems to be the encouragement behind the beatitude "Blessed are those who mourn . . ."

6. Adapted from the module on vulnerability in Karen Anderson and Gert Rüppell, *Facing AIDS: Education in the Context of Vulnerability* (Geneva: WCC Publications, 1999), http://hivhealthclearinghouse.unesco.org/sites/default/files/resources/bie_world_council_churches_facing_aids_en.pdf.

7. Elizabeth Knox-Seith, ed., *One Body: North-South Reflections in the Face of HIV and AIDS* (Copenhagen: The Nordic-Foccisa Church Cooperation, 2005), http://www.norgeskristnerad.no/doc//One%20Body/OneBody-vol1-Eng.pdf.

8. Musa W. Dube, "Let There Be Light! Birthing Ecumenical Theology in the HIV and AIDS Apocalypse," 2014 Niblett Memorial Lecture, Sarum College, Salisbury, UK, published in *The Ecumenical Review* 67, no. 4 (December 2015): 531–42.

9. Adriaan S. van Klinken, "When the Body of Christ Has AIDS: A Theological Metaphor for Global Solidarity in Light of HIV & AIDS," *International Journal of Public Theology* 4 (2010): 446–65.

10. Statement on "HIV-positive Theology," from the consultation "The Body of Christ Is HIV-positive?" 13–17 June 2011, Birmingham, UK, in Gideon Byamugisha, John J. Raja, and Ezra Chitando, eds., *Is the Body of Christ HIV-positive? New Ecclesiological Christologies in the Context of HIV-positive Communities* (New Delhi/Birmingham: ISPCK/ SOCMS, 2012), 238–41.

11. Adapted from Maxwell Lawton's web site, http://www.maxwelllawton.com/abouttheartist.html.

12. "Churches' Compassionate Response to HIV and AIDS," statement by the WCC Central Committee, Geneva, 6 September 2006, https://www.oikoumene.org/en/resources/documents/commissions/international-affairs/human-rights-and-impunity/churches-compassionate-response-to-hiv-and-aids.

13. WCC, *Facing AIDS: The Challenge, The Churches' Response*, a WCC Study Document (Geneva: WCC Publications, 1997).

14. Adapted and developed from Nyambura Njoroge's "Follow Me: Marching Orders from Above!" in Byamugisha, et al., eds., *Is the Body of Christ HIV-positive?* 3–11.

15. Musa W. Dube, ed., *AfricaPraying: A Handbook on HIV/AIDS Sensitive Sermons and Liturgy* (Geneva: WCC Publications, 2003), https://www.oikoumene.org/en/folder/documents-pdf/africa-praying-eng.pdf.

16. Pontifical Council for Promoting Christian Unity/The Commission on Faith and Order of the World Council of Churches, "Resources for The Week of Prayer for Christian Unity and throughout the year 2007," http://www.vatican.va/roman_curia/pontifical_councils/chrstuni/weeks-prayer-doc/rc_pc_chrstuni_doc_20060703_week-prayer-2007_en.html.

17. The Ujamaa Centre for Biblical and Theological Community Development and Research, based at the University of Kwazulu-Natal, Pietermaritzburg, emerged in a time of deep conflict in the KwaZulu-Natal region of South Africa. The struggles against apartheid in KwaZulu-Natal in the late 1980s brought socially engaged biblical scholars, organic intellectuals, and displaced communities into daily contact. The Centre hosted the reading of the Bible together, taking seriously the contributions of each other. "Contextual Bible Study" emerged out of this process. The Contextual Bible Study of Tamar's rape (2 Sam. 13:12-18) was developed in 1996 and eventually developed into the Tamar Campaign.

18. Ted Karpf and Alex Ross, eds., *Building from Common Foundations: The World Health Organization and Faith-Based Organizations in Primary Health-care* (Geneva: World Health Organization, 2008), http://apps.who.int/iris/bitstr eam/10665/43884/1/9789241596626_eng.pdf.

19. An overview of the history, members, and main activities of the Christian Health Associations may be found in Franck Dimmock, Jill Olivier, and Quentin Wodon, "Half a Century Young: The Christian Health Associations in Africa," MPRA Paper No. 45369, March 2013, http://mpra.ub.uni-muenchen.de/45369/.

20. WCC, "Human Resource Challenges in Faith-Based Organizations," *Contact* 190 (Winter/Spring 2011), https://www.oikoumene.org/en/what-we-do/health-and-healing/CONTACT190.pdf.

21. ACHAP HIV/AIDS technical working group: http://africachap.org/en/hiv-aids/.

22. EPN, *HIV/AIDS Treatment Literacy Guide for Church Leaders/Guide de formation sur le traitement du VIH SIDA pour les leaders d'Eglises* (Nairobi: Ecumenical Pharmaceutical Network, 2010).

Chapter 3: Living with HIV

1. UNAIDS, *On the Fast-Track to End AIDS by 2030: Focus on Location and Population* (Geneva: UNAIDS, 2015), http://www.unaids.org/sites/default/files/media_asset/WAD2015_report_en_part01.pdf.

2. A. L. Stangl, et al., "A Systematic Review of Interventions to Reduce HIV-Related Stigma and Discrimination from 2002 to 2013: How Far Have We Come?" *Journal of the International AIDS Society* 16, Supplement 2 (13 November 2013): 18734.

3. I. T. Katz, et al., "Impact of HIV-Related Stigma on Treatment Adherence: Systematic Review and Meta-synthesis" *Journal of the International AIDS Society* 16, Supplement 2 (13 November 2013): 18640.

4. The People Living with HIV Stigma Index provides a tool that measures and detects changing trends in relation to stigma and discrimination experienced by people living with HIV; http://www.stigmaindex.org/.

5. UNAIDS, *On the Fast-Track* (see n.1, above).

6. R. C. Dellar, et al., "Adolescent Girls and Young Women: Key Populations for HIV Epidemic Control," *Journal of the International AIDS Society* 18, Supplement 1 (26 February 2015): 19408.

7. Referring to gays and lesbians, homosexuals, or men who have sex with men.

8. Linus Bengtsson, "Global HIV Surveillance among MSM: Is Risk Behaviour Seriously Underestimated?" *Journal of the International AIDS Society* 24, no. 15 (24 September 2010): 2301–2303, http://journals.lww.com/aidsonline/Fulltext/2010/09240/Global_HIV_surveillance_among_MSM__is_risk.1.aspx.

9. The Global Fund, "Addressing Sex Work, MSM & Transgender People in the Context of the HIV Epidemic," 2011, http://asapltd.com/wp-content/uploads/2013/07/Core_SOGI_InfoNote_en.pdf.

10. More information on the AIDS quilt may be found at http://www.aidsquilt.org/about/the-aids-memorial-quilt.

11. AIDSFOCUS, "Memory Work," http://www.aidsfocus.ch/en/topics-and-resources/prevention-treatment-and-care/memory-work.

12. Sinomlando, "Memory Work," http://sinomlando.ukzn.ac.za/index.php/en/memory-work-mainmenu-47

13. Adapted from Ernesto Barroso Cardoso, "The Experience of Faith in the Face of Suffering . . . ," in WCC, *Facing AIDS: The Challenge, the Churches' Response*, a WCC Study Document (Geneva: WCC Publications, 1997), 35–43, http://wcc-coe.org/wcc/what/mission/ehaia-pdf/facing-aids-eng.pdf.

14. Adapted from a quote by Ernesto Barroso Cardoso, in Maren C. Tirabassi and Kathy Wonson Eddy, eds., *Gifts of Many Cultures: Worship Resources for the Global Community* (Cleveland: United Church Press, 1995), 4.

15. Jim Wooten, *We Are All the Same: A Story of a Boy's Courage and a Mother's Love* (New York: Penguin, 2005).

16. Elie Wiesel, *Night*, a new trans. by Marion Wiesel (New York: Hill and Wang, 2006), 65 (originally written in Yiddish; first published in French, Paris: Les Editions de Minuit, 1958).

17. The Nobel Peace Prize acceptance speech delivered by Elie Wiesel in Oslo on 10 December 1986, in ibid., 117–20.

18. Robert Igo, O.S.B., "Making Sense of Suffering," in Igo, *A Window into Hope: An Invitation to Faith in the Context of HIV/AIDS* (Geneva: WCC Publications, 2009), 121–44

19. Gideon Byamugisha and Glen Williams, eds., *Positive Voices: Religious Leaders Living with or Personally Affected by HIV and AIDS*, Called to Care (Oxford: Strategies for Hope Trust, 2005).

20. John W. Ayers, Benjamin M. Althouse, Mark Dredze, Eric C. Leas, and Seth M. Noar, "News and Internet Searches about Human Immunodeficiency Virus after Charlie Sheen's Disclosure," *Journal of the American Medical Association Internal Medicine* (22 February 2016), http://archinte.jamanetwork.com/article.aspx?articleid=2495274#ild160001r4.

21. The SAVE Toolkit may be found at http://inerela.org/resources/save-toolkit/.

22. Adapted from "A Discussion with Rev. Canon Gideon Byamugisha," 3 May 2009, Georgetown University—Berkley Centre for Religion, Peace, and World Affairs, http://berkleycenter.georgetown.edu/interviews/a-discussion-with-rev-canon-gideon-byamugisha-founder-african-network-of-religious-leaders-living-with-or-personally-affected-by-hiv-aids.

23. Rev. Fr J. P. Mokgethi-Heath, in Geneva, on 2 November 2015, speaking at the discussion on the book *Dignity, Freedom, and Grace: Christian Perspectives on HIV, AIDS, and Human Rights*, ed. Gillian Paterson and Callie Long (Geneva: WCC Publications, 2016).

24. Adapted from Gracia Violeta Ross Quiroga, "Thoughts and Reflections on the Theme: 'God, in Your Grace, Transform our Witness,'" in Luis N. Rivera-Pagán, ed., *God, in Your Grace: Official Report of the Ninth Assembly of the World Council of Churches* (Geneva: WCC Publications, 2007), 102–111.

25. Interview with Gracia Violeta Ross Quiroga by Manoj Kurian, 26 February 2016.

26. R. K. Kambodji and S. Jacob, *Journey of Life: Living, Not Just Existing, Stories of Brothers/Sisters Living with HIV* (Hong Kong: Christian Conference of Asia, 2013), 55–67.

27. UNAIDS, "The Denver Principles," 1983, http://data.unaids.org/pub/ExternalDocument/2007/gipa1983denverprinciples_en.pdf.

28. The Framework for Dialogue may be found at http://www.frameworkfordia-logue.net/.

Chapter 4: Safe Spaces of Grace

1. Adapted from the module on vulnerability in Karen Anderson and Gert Rüppell, *Facing AIDS: Education in the Context of Vulnerability* (Geneva: WCC Publications, 1999), http://hivhealthclearinghouse.unesco.org/sites/default/files/resources/bie_world_council_churches_facing_aids_en.pdf.

2. "And about three o'clock Jesus cried with a loud voice, '*Eli, Eli, lema sabachthani?*' that is, 'My God, my God, why have you forsaken me?'"

3. Developed from "Six features of supportive social spaces," suggested by Catherine Campbell, Morten Skovdal, and Andrew Gibbs in "Creating Social Spaces to Tackle AIDS-Related Stigma: Reviewing the Role of Church Groups in Sub-Saharan Africa," *AIDS and Behavior* 15, no. 6 (August 2011): 1204–19, http://uib.academia.edu/MortenSkovdal/Papers/199897/Creating_social_spaces_to_tackle_AIDS-related_stigma_Reviewing_the_role_of_Church_groups_in_sub-Saharan_Africa.

4. Rick James, *Creating Space for Grace: God's Power in Organisational Change* (Sundbyberg: Swedish Mission Council, 2004), http://www.prismaweb.org/media/196134/04_02_space_for_grace.pdf.

5. Musa W. Dube, ed., *HIV/AIDS and the Curriculum: Methods of Integrating HIV/AIDS in Theological Programmes* (Geneva: WCC Publications, 2003).

6. Ezra Chitando, ed., *Mainstreaming HIV and AIDS in Theological Education: Experiences and Explorations*, EHAIA (Geneva: WCC Publications, 2008).

7. Rachael C. Dellar, Sarah Diamini, and Quarraisha Abdool Karim, "Adolescent Girls and Young Women: Key Populations for HIV Epidemic Control," *Journal of the International AIDS Society* 18, Supplement 1 (26 February 2015): 19408, http://www.jiasociety.org/index.php/jias/article/view/19408

8. UNAIDS, *The GAP Report*, 2014, http://www.unaids.org/sites/default/files/media_asset/UNAIDS_Gap_report_en.pdf.

9. World YWCA, *Reclaiming and Redefining Rights: ICPD+20: Status of Sexual and Reproductive Health and Rights in Africa*, Monitoring Report, April 2013 (Geneva: World YWCA, 2013), http://arrow.org.my/wp-content/uploads/2015/04/ICPD-20-Africa_Monitoring-Report_2013.pdf.

10. World YWCA, "African Union Girl Summit on Ending Child Marriage in Africa," 24 November 2015, http://www.worldywca.org/YWCA-News/World-YWCA-and-Member-Associations-News/African-Union-Girl-Summit-on-ending-child-marriage-in-Africa.

11. Ezra Chitando and Nontando Hadebe, eds., *Compassionate Circles: African Women Theologians Facing HIV* (Geneva: WCC Publications, 2009).

12. From personal communication with Dr. Isabel Phiri.

13. Eric Y. Tenkorang, "Marriage, Widowhood, Divorce and HIV Risks among Women in Sub-Saharan Africa," *International Health* 6, no. 1 (2014): 46–53.

14. Interview with Reverend Phumzile Zondi-Mabizela, executive director, INERELA+, 24 February 2016.

15. Brian Perry, et al., "Widow Cleansing and Inheritance among the Luo in Kenya: The Need for Additional Women-centred HIV Prevention Options," *Journal of the International AIDS Society* 17 (26 June 2014): 19010, http://www.jiasociety.org/index.php/jias/article/view/19010.

16. Adapted from the section "Violence against Women," in Musa W. Dube, ed., *Africa Praying: A Handbook on HIV/AIDS Sensitive Sermons and Liturgy* (Geneva: WCC Publications, 2003).

17. Myra Betron, Gary Barker, Juan Manual Contreras, and Dean Peacock, *Men, Masculinities and HIV/AIDS: Strategies for Action* (Washington, DC: International Center for Research on Women/Rio de Janeiro: Instituto Promundo/Cape Town: MenEngage Alliance and Sonke Gender Justice Network, 2008), http://www.genderjustice.org.za/publication/men-masculinities-hivaids/.

18. Adriaan Van Klinken and Ezra Chitando, "Masculinities, HIV and Religion in Africa," in Emma Tomalin, ed., *The Routledge Handbook of Religions and Global Development* (New York and London: Routledge, 2015), 127–37.

19. REDLACTRANS and International AIDS Alliance, "The Night Is Another Country: Impunity and Violence against Transgender Women Human Rights Defenders in Latin America" (Buenos Aires: REDLACTRANS/Hove, UK: International AIDS Alliance, 2013), http://www.aidsalliance.org/resources/302-the-night-is-another-country.

20. Stefan D. Baral, et al., "Worldwide Burden of HIV in Transgender Women: A Systematic Review and Meta-analysis," *The Lancet–Infectious Diseases* 13, no. 3 (March 2013): 214–22.

21. L. William Countryman, *Dirt, Greed and Sex: Sexual Ethics in the New Testament and Their Implications for Today* (Minneapolis: Fortress Press, 1989).

22. John Riches, *Jesus and the Transformation of Judaism* (London: Darton, Longman & Todd, 1980).

23. Beverley G. Haddad, "'We Pray but We Cannot Heal': Theological Challenges Posed by the HIV/AIDS Crisis," *Journal of Theology for South Africa* 125 (July 2006): 80–90.

24. Rev. Dr Samuel Kobia, WCC General Secretary, "Letter to the Uganda President Yoweri Kaguta Museveni, 'Raising Concerns regarding Anti Homosexuality Bill, 2009,'" 22 December 2009, http://www.oikoumene.org/en/resources/documents/general-secretary/messages-and-letters/letter-to-the-uganda-president.html.

25. Manoj Kurian, "An Ecumenical Framework for a Liberative Human Sexuality: Toward a Culture of Justice and Peace," *Ecumenical Review* 64, no. 3 (October 2012): 338–45.

26. For example, the United Church of Christ in the Philippines, National Council of Churches in the Philippines, National Council of Churches in India, and Latin American Council of Churches (CLAI).

27. WCC-EHAIA, "Dealing as a Church with HIV," 13 October 2014, https://www.oikoumene.org/en/press-centre/news/dealing-as-a-church-with-hiv.

28. From a posting by George Barasa on the Facebook page of Kuchu Times Kenyan Correspondent-Jojibaro, 20 June 2013, https://www.facebook.com/permalink.php?story_fbid=586519141380070&id=561735000525151.

29. A large number of churches and denominational and ecumenical bodies, including the WCC, are members of the "We Will Speak Out" coalition, http://www.wewillspeakout.org/.

30. At the time of this dialogue in 2012, Rowan Williams was the Archbishop of Canterbury and Michel Sidibé the executive director of UNAIDS. Adapted from "More than a Prayer: Faith Communities' Response to Sexual Violence: A Dialogue between Archbishop Rowan Williams and Michel Sidibé of UNAIDS for World AIDS Day," 30 November 2012, http://www.newstatesman.com/lifestyle/2012/11/more-prayer-faith-communities-response-sexual-violence.

31. UNWomen, "Church Bells Ring for Women and Girls," 8 October 2013, http://www.unwomen.org/en/news/stories/2013/10/in-ethiopia-church-bells-ring-for-women-and-girls.

32. Gerald West and Phumzile Zondi-Mabezela, "The Bible Story That Became a Campaign: The Tamar Campaign in South Africa (and Beyond)," *Ministerial Formation* 103 (July 2004): 4–12, http://ujamaa.ukzn.ac.za/Files/the bible story.pdf.

33. Ezra Chitando and Sophie Chirongoma, eds., *Redemptive Masculinities: Men, HIV, and Religion* (Geneva: WCC Publications, 2012).

Chapter 5: Walk the Walk, Talk the Talk

1. John H. Bryant, "Principles of Justice as a Basis for Conceptualizing a Health Care System," *International Journal of Health Services* 7 (1977): 707–719.

2. James C. McGilvray, *The Quest for Health and Wholeness* (Tübingen: German Institute for Medical Mission, 1981).

3. Ezra Chitando, *Living with Hope: African Churches and HIV/AIDS* 1 (Geneva: WCC Publications, 2007), 2.

4. "Contre les violences sexuelles à l'égard des filles," *Togo-Presse* n° 9729-du 17/022016-page 8.

5. Personal correspondence with Ms. Ayoko Bahun-Wilson, regional coordinator for West Africa, WCC-EHAIA.

6. Barbara Schmid, Elizabeth Thomas, Jill Olivier, and James R. Cochrane, *The Contribution of Religious Entities to Health in Sub-Saharan Africa*, an ARHAP Report, May 2008 (Cape Town: African Religious Health Assets Programme [ARHAP], 2008), https://docs.google.com/viewerng/viewer?url=http://jliflc.com/wp-content/uploads/2014/08/ARHAPGates_full.pdf.

7. PEPFAR, *A Firm Foundation: The PEPFAR Consultation on the Role of Faith-Based Organizations in Sustaining Community and Country Leadership in the Response to HIV/AIDS* (Washington, DC: U.S. Department of State, 2012), http://www.pepfar.gov/documents/organization/195614.pdf.

8. CARITAS Internationalis, "Caritas Is Church," http://www.caritas.org/who-we-are/caritas-church/.

9. World Vision International, "HIV and AIDS Programmes: World Vision's HIV and AIDS Response," http://www.wvi.org/health/hiv-and-aids-programmes.

10. WCC-EAA, "Live the Promise: HIV Campaign," https://www.oikoumene.org/en/what-we-do/eaa/live-the-promise-hiv-campaign.

Chapter 6: Visions of the Future

1. Viviane D. Lima, Lillian Lourenço, Benita Yip, Robert S. Hogg, Peter Phillips, and Julio S. G. Montaner, "AIDS Incidence and AIDS-Related Mortality in British Columbia, Canada, between 1981 and 2013: A retrospective study," *The Lancet HIV* 2, no. 3 (March 2015): 92–97, http://dx.doi.org/10.1016/S2352-3018(15)00017-X.

2. UNAIDS, *Global Report: UNAIDS Report on the Global AIDS Epidemic 2013* (Geneva: UNAIDS, 2013), http://www.unaids.org/sites/default/files/media_asset/UNAIDS_Global_Report_2013_en_1.pdf.

3. UNAIDS, "Fast-Track: Ending the AIDS Epidemic by 2030," 2014, http://www.unaids.org/en/resources/documents/2014/JC2686_WAD2014report.

4. Roger Ying, Ruanne V. Barnabas, and Brian G. Williams, "Modeling the Implementation of Universal Coverage for HIV Treatment as Prevention and Its Impact on the HIV Epidemic," *Current HIV/AIDS Reports* 11 (2014): 459–67, http://www.ncbi.nlm.nih.gov/pmc/articles/PMC4301303/.

5. "The HIV treatment continuum—sometimes also referred to as the HIV care cascade—is a model that outlines the sequential steps or stages of HIV medical care that people living with HIV go through from initial diagnosis to achieving the goal of viral suppression (a very low level of HIV in the body), and shows the proportion of individuals living with HIV who are engaged at each stage. In 2011, Dr. Edward Gardner and colleagues observed that 'for individuals with HIV to fully benefit from potent combination antiretroviral therapy, they need to know that they are HIV infected, be engaged in regular HIV care, and receive and adhere to effective antiretroviral therapy.' They acknowledged, however, that various obstacles contribute to poor engagement in HIV care, substantially limiting the effectiveness of efforts to improve health outcomes for those with HIV and to reduce new HIV transmissions. So, the researchers set out to describe and quantify the spectrum of engagement in HIV care. The result of the researchers' work was the HIV care continuum (or 'cascade'), which they defined as having the following stages: diagnosis of HIV infection, linkage to care, retention in care, receipt of antiretroviral therapy, and achievement of viral suppression." HIV/AIDS Care Continuum, https://www.aids.gov/federal-resources/policies/care-continuum/.

6. UNAIDS, "Fast-Track" (see n.3 above).

7. The team used a model to calculate the funding the countries will need to 2050, based on four different scenarios, with data from a publicly available UNAIDS tool called Spectrum.

8. "Front-loading" is defined as changing the phasing of a program so that it uses the same total inputs, but uses them more quickly so that outputs are realized sooner. Predictable and front-loaded spending, as opposed to spending the same resources year to year, can affect HIV-care programming and health benefits.

9. Rifat Atun, et al., "Long-Term Financing Needs for HIV Control in Sub-Saharan Africa in 2015–2050: A modelling study," *BMJ Open* 6, no. 3 (6 March 2016), http://bmjopen.bmj.com/content/6/3/e009656.abstract.

10. Stefano Vella, "End of AIDS on the Horizon, but Innovation Needed to End HIV," *The Lancet HIV* 2, no. 3 (March 2015): e74–e75,

11. UNAIDS, "The GAP Report," 2014, http://www.unaids.org/sites/default/files/media_asset/UNAIDS_Gap_report_en.pdf.

12. "Do not judge, so that you may not be judged" (Matt. 7:1).

13. Rachael C. Dellar, Sarah Dlamini, and Quarraisha Abdool Karim, "Adolescent Girls and Young Women: Key Populations for HIV Epidemic Control," *Journal of the International AIDS Society* 18, Supplement 1 (2015): 19408, http://www.jiasociety.org/index.php/jias/article/view/19408.

14. Brot für die Welt, Christian AID, DanChurchAID, FinnChurchAID, ICCO, Kerk in Actie, and Norwegian Church AIDS, *Human Rights, HIV/AIDS Prevention, and Gender Equality: An Impossible Cocktail for Faith Based Organisations?* Position Paper, 2008, http://www.bibalex.org/Search4Dev/document/283610.

15. World YWCA, "YWCA Safe Spaces for Women and Girls: A Global Model for Change, Mobilising Young Women Leadership on SRHR and HIV," 2014,

http://www.worldywca.org/Resources/YWCA-Publications/YWCA-Safe-Spaces-for-Women-and-Girls-A-Global-Model-for-Change.

16. UNAIDS, *Global Report: Report on the Global AIDS Epidemic* (Geneva: UNAIDS, 2012), http://www.unaids.org/en/media/unaids/contentassets/documents/epidemiology/2012/gr2012/20121120_UNAIDS_Global_Report_2012_with_annexes_en.pdf.

17. Daniel Wolfe and Kasia Malinowska-Sempruch, "Illicit Drug Policies and the Global HIV Epidemic: Effects of UN and National Government Approaches," A working paper commissioned by the HIV/AIDS Task Force of the Millennium Project 2004 (New York: Open Society Institute, 2004), https://www.opensocietyfoundations.org/reports/illicit-drug-policies-and-global-hiv-epidemic.

18. Bradley M. Mathers, Louisa Degenhardt, and Benjamin Phillips, et al., "Global Epidemiology of Injecting Drug Use and HIV among People Who Inject Drugs: A Systematic Review," *The Lancet* 372, no. 9561 (2008): 1733–45, http://www.ncbi.nlm.nih.gov/pubmed/18817968.

19. Naloxone is a medication used to block or reverse the effects of opioid medication, including extreme drowsiness, slowed breathing, or loss of consciousness. An opioid is sometimes called a narcotic.

20. Joanne Csete, M.D., et al., "Public Health and International Drug Policy," *The Lancet* 387, no. 10026 (2 April 2016): 1427–80, http://www.thelancet.com/journals/lancet/article/PIIS0140-6736%2816%2900619-X/abstract.

21. World Health Organization, "WHO: People Most at Risk of HIV Are Not Getting the Health Services They Need," 11 July 2014, http://www.who.int/mediacentre/news/releases/2014/key-populations-to-hiv/en/.

22. Chris Beyrer, et al., "Global Epidemiology of HIV Infection in Men Who Have Sex with Men," *The Lancet* 380, no. 9839 (28 July 2012): 367–77, http://www.thelancet.com/journals/lancet/article/PIIS0140-6736%2812%2960821-6/abstract.

23. Chris Beyrer, et al., "A Call to Action for Comprehensive HIV Services for Men Who Have Sex with Men," *The Lancet* 380, no. 9839 (28 July 2012): 424–38, http://www.thelancet.com/journals/lancet/article/PIIS0140-6736%2812%2961022-8/abstract.

24. Anette Agardh, et al., "Health Risks in Same-Sex Attracted Ugandan University Students: Evidence from Two Cross-Sectional Studies," PLOS ONE, 11, no. 3 (16 March 2016): e0150627, http://journals.plos.org/plosone/article?id=10.1371/journal.pone.0150627.

25. Lucas Paoli Itabora and Jingshu Zhu, "State-Sponsored Homophobia: A World Survey on Laws: Criminalization, Protection and Respect of Same-Sex Love," May 2014, 9th ed. (Geneva: ILGA, 2014), http://old.ilga.org/Statehomophobia/ILGA_SSHR_2014_Eng.pdf.

26. Homophobia is the irrational fear of, aversion to, or discrimination against homosexuality or homosexuals.

27. Transphobia is a range of antagonistic attitudes and feelings against transsexuality and transsexual or transgender people.

28. Donald P. McNeill, Douglas A. Morrison, and Henri J. M. Nouwen, *Compassion: A Reflection on the Christian Life* (New York: Doubleday/Image Books, 1982), 3–4.

29. Interview with Gracia Violeta Ross Quiroga, 24 February 2016.

30. WCC, "Churches and Agencies Formulate Responses to Ebola Outbreak," 1 October 2014, http://www.oikoumene.org/en/press-centre/news/churches-and-agencies-formulate-responses-to-ebola-outbreak.

31. Mark A. Wainberg, Susan Kippax, Marlène Bras, and Papa S. Sow, "HIV and Ebola: Similarities and Differences," *Journal of the International AIDS Society* 17, no.1 (1 December 2014): 19896, http://www.jiasociety.org/index.php/jias/article/view/19896.

32. WCC, "Churches and Agencies Formulate Responses to Ebola Outbreak" (see n. 30, above).

33. World Health Organization, "New WHO Safe and Dignified Burial Protocol—Key to Reducing Ebola Transmission," 7 November 2014, http://www.who.int/mediacentre/news/notes/2014/ebola-burial-protocol/en/.

34. WCC, "Ecumenical Ebola Response," Newsletter no. 3 (27 February 2015), https://www.oikoumene.org/en/what-we-do/health-and-healing/ebola-newsletter/newsletter-ndeg-3-27-february-2015.

35. WHO, "Hepatitis C," Fact Sheet No. 164 (July 2015), http://www.who.int/mediacentre/factsheets/fs164/en/.

36. Roger D. Kouyos, et al., "Clustering of HCV Coinfection on HIV Phylogeny Indicates Domestic and Sexual Transmission of HCV," *International Journal of Epidemiology* 43, no. 3 (June 2014): 887–96.

37. TreatASIA/AMFAR, "Hepatitis C Treatment Snapshots: Sofosbuvir," August 2015, http://www.amfar.org/uploadedFiles/_amfarorg/Around_the_World/TREAT_Asia/TA_Snapshots_Hep_C_080515.pdf.

38. Gareth J. Owen, "The Hierarchical Experience of Stigma in HIV/Hepatitis C Co-Infected Gay Men," in Pranee Liamputtong, ed., *Stigma, Discrimination, and Living with HIV/AIDS: A Cross-Cultural Perspective* (New York: Springer, 2013), 309–322.

Historical Timeline

1. Apart from ecumenical sources, adapted from the following sources:
   - AMFAR, "Thirty Years of HIV/AIDS: Snapshots of an Epidemic," http://www.amfar.org/thirty-years-of-hiv/aids-snapshots-of-an-epidemic/.
   - AVERT, "History of HIV and AIDS Overview," http://www.avert.org/professionals/history-hiv-aids/overview.
   - AIDS.gov, "A Timeline of HIV/AIDS," https://www.aids.gov/hiv-aids-basics/hiv-aids-101/aids-timeline/.
   - International AIDS Society, "History of International AIDS Conferences," http://www.aids2014.org/webcontent/file/History_of_the_International_AIDS_Conference.pdf.

2. David Serwadda, et al., "Slim Disease: A New Disease in Uganda and Its Association with HTLV-III Infection," *The Lancet* 326, no. 8460 (1985): 849–52.

3. Françoise Barré-Sinoussi, et al., "Isolation of a T-lymphotropic Retrovirus from a Patient at Risk for Acquired Immune Deficiency Syndrome (AIDS)," *Science* 220, no. 4599 (20 May 1983): 868–71.

Bibliography

WCC, Ecumenical, and Church-Related Publications

Ackermann, Denise. *Tamar's Cry: Re-reading an Ancient Text in the Midst of an HIV/AIDS Pandemic.* Changing Minds, Changing Lives. Stellenbosch: EFSA, 2001. Rev. ed.: London: Catholic Institute for International Relations, 2002.

Anderson, Karen, and Gert Rüppell. *Facing AIDS: Education in the Context of Vulnerability.* Study Guide accompanying the World Council of Churches' Study Document on HIV/AIDS, *Facing Aids: The Challenge, the Churches Response.* Geneva: WCC Publications, 1999. http://hivhealthclearinghouse.unesco.org/sites/default/files/resources/bie_world_council_churches_facing_aids_en.pdf.

Almedal, Calle. "A Thirty-Year Personal Journey with HIV." *The Ecumenical Review* 63, no. 4 (December 2011): 369–77.

Azetsop, Jacquineau, ed. *HIV and AIDS in Africa: Christian Reflection, Public Health, Social Transformation.* Maryknoll, NY: Orbis, 2016.

Backlund, Charlotte, Karl-Erik Lundgren, Lena Boberg, Lorentz Forsberg, and Rick James. *The OD Booklet: Useful Models and Practices in Organisational Development.* Sundbyberg: Swedish Mission Council (SMC), 2007. http://www.missioncouncil.se/wp/wp-content/uploads/2011/05/The_OD_Booklet.pdf.

Bayley, Anne, and Mugrove Walter Nyika. *More and Better Food: Farming, Climate Change, Health and the AIDS epidemic.* Called to Care series. Oxford: Strategies for Hope Trust, 2011.

Benn, Christoph, and Erlinda Senturias. "Health, Healing and Wholeness in the Ecumenical Discussion." *International Review of Mission* 90, nos. 356/357 (2001): 7–25.

Berner-Rodoreda, Astrid. *HIV in Africa: A Female Epidemic Requiring Only a Female Response? The Gender Dimension of HIV and AIDS in Africa and Good Practice Examples from Partner Organisations of Bread for the World.* Stuttgart: Brot für die Welt, 2008.

———, and Carsta Neuenroth. *The Burden of Breadwinning: Transformative Masculinities in the Context of HIV, Violence against Women and Gender Inequality.* Dialogue 17: Practice. Stuttgart: Brot für die Welt, 2016.

Breetvelt, Jaap, ed. *Theological Responses to the HIV and AIDS Pandemic.* GIRO 456. Utrecht: Kerk in Actie, 2009. http://www.luisterenddienen.nl/site/uploadedDocs/Theologicalresponseshivaids.pdf.

Brot für die Welt, Christian AID, DanChurchAID, FinnChurchAID, ICCO, Kerk in Actie, Norwegian Church AIDS. *Human Rights, HIV/AIDS Prevention, and Gender Equality: An Impossible Cocktail for Faith Based Organisations?* Position Paper. 2008. http://www.bibalex.org/Search4Dev/document/283610.

Byamugisha, Gideon, and Glen Williams, eds. *Positive Voices: Religious Leaders Living with or Personally Affected by HIV and AIDS.* Called to Care series. Oxford: Strategies for Hope Trust, 2005.

Carman, Lucy, and Pippa Durn. *Keep the Promise: A Teaching Resource on Advocacy and HIV and AIDS.* Geneva: Ecumenical Advocacy Alliance, 2006. http://www.e-alliance.ch/en/s/hivaids/keep-the-promise/index.html.

Christian Aid and Strategies for Hope. *What Can I Do? The HIV/AIDS Ministry and Messages of Canon Gideon Byamugisha.* DVD. 49 min. 2004. http://www.stratshope.org/resources/dvds_item/what-can-i-do.

———. "A Facilitator's Guide to *What Can I Do?*" Oxford: Strategies for Hope Trust, 2004. Available in English, French, Portuguese, Spanish and Swahili.

Chitando, Ezra. *Living with Hope: African Churches and HIV/AIDS* 1. Geneva: WCC Publications, 2007.

———. *Acting in Hope: African Churches and HIV/AIDS* 2. Geneva: WCC Publications, 2007.

———, ed. *Mainstreaming HIV and AIDS in Theological Education: Experiences and Explorations.* EHAIA series. Geneva: WCC Publications, 2008.

———, ed. *Troubled but Not Destroyed: African Theology in Dialogue with HIV and AIDS.* Geneva: WCC Publications, 2009.

———, and Nontando Hadebe, eds. *Compassionate Circles: African Women Theologians Facing HIV.* Geneva: WCC Publications, 2009.

_____, and Sophie Chirongoma, eds. *Redemptive Masculinities: Men, HIV, and Religion.* Geneva: WCC Publications, 2012.

_____, and Nyambura J. Njoroge, eds. *Transformative Masculinity: Contextual Bible Study Manual.* Harare: WCC/EHAIA, 2013.

Cimperman, Maria. *When God's People Have AIDS: An Approach to Ethics.* Maryknoll, NY: Orbis, 2006.

Davila, Emily. *Faith Advocacy Toolkit: Advocacy for Universal Access: A Toolkit for Faith-Based Organisations.* Geneva: Ecumenical Advocacy Alliance, 2008. http://repository.berkleycenter.georgetown.edu/100101EcumenicalAdvocacyAllianceFaithAdvocacyToolkit.pdf.

Doupe, Andrew. *Partnerships between Churches and People Living with HIV/AIDS Organizations: Guidelines.* Geneva: WCC Publications, 2005.

_____. "Working with People Living with HIV/AIDS Organizations." Background Document. Geneva: WCC, 2005.

Dube, Musa W. "Preaching to the Converted: Unsettling the Christian Church." *Ministerial Formation* 93 (2001b): 38–50.

_____, ed. *Africa Praying: A Handbook on HIV/AIDS Sensitive Sermons and Liturgy.* Geneva: WCC Publications, 2003. https://www.oikoumene.org/en/folder/documents-pdf/africa-praying-eng.pdf.

_____, ed. *HIV/AIDS and the Curriculum: Methods of Integrating HIV/AIDS in Theological Programmes.* Geneva: WCC Publications, 2003.

_____, series ed. *Module 4: Reading the New Testament in the HIV & AIDS Contexts.* Theology in the HIV & AID Era series. HIV & AIDS Curriculum For Theological Education by Extension Programmes and Institutions. Geneva: WCC Publications, 2007. https://www.oikoumene.org/en/resources/documents/wcc-programmes/justice-diakonia-and-responsibility-for-creation/ehaia/trainingteaching-material/EHAIA_TEE_Module_04.pdf.

Evangelical Church in Germany (EKD). "For a Life with Dignity: The Global Threat of HIV/AIDS: Possible Courses of Action for the Church." A Study by the Evangelical Church in Germany's Advisory Commission on Sustainable Development. EKD Texts 91. Hanover: 2007. https://www.ekd.de/english/download/aids_text_91.pdf.

Gennrich, Daniela, et al. *Created in God's Image: A Gender Transformation Toolkit for Women and Men in Churches.* Rev. ed. Oslo/Pretoria: Norwegian Church AID, 2008, 2013. https://www.kirkensnodhjelp.no/contentassets/c2cd7731ab1b4727897258c5d49246c8/nca-createdingodsimage-completebook-jun2015-open2.pdf.

Igo, Robert, O.S.B. *Listening with Love: Pastoral Counselling—A Christian Response to People Living with HIV/AIDS.* Geneva: WCC Publications,

2005. https://www.oikoumene.org/en/folder/documents-pdf/listening-withlove-e.pdf.

———. *A Window into Hope: An Invitation to Faith in the Context of HIV and AIDS.* Geneva: WCC Publications, 2009.

INERELA+. "SAVE Toolkit." 2012. http://inerela.org/resources/resourcessave-toolkit-second-edition/.

James, Rick. *Creating Space for Grace: God's Power in Organisational Change.* Sundbyberg: Swedish Mission Council, 2004. http://www.prismaweb.org/media/196134/04_02_space_for_grace.pdf.

Kambodji, R. K., and S. Jacob. *Journey of Life: Living, Not Just Existing, Stories of Brothers/Sisters Living with HIV.* Hong Kong: Christian Conference of Asia, 2013.

———, E. N. Senturias, and A.W. Longchar, eds. *HIV and Inclusive Community: Asian Theological and Biblical Perspectives.* Hong Kong: Christian Conference of Asia, 2013.

Klagba, Charles, and C. B. Peter, eds. *Into the Sunshine: Integrating HIV/AIDS in the Ethics Curriculum.* Geneva: WCC Publications, 2005.

Knox-Seith, Elizabeth, ed. *One Body—AIDS and the Worshipping Community: Bible Studies, Liturgies and Personal Stories from South and North.* Oslo: The Nordic-Foccisa Church Cooperation, 2005. http://www.norgeskristnerad.no/doc/One%20Body/OneBody-Vol2%20-Eng.pdf.

———, and Reuben Daka, eds. *One Body: Human Dignity Inherent in Every Human Being: Towards Gender Equality, including Young People and Overcoming Abuse.* Oslo: The Nordic-Foccisa Church Cooperation, 2014. http://www.norgeskristnerad.no/doc/One%20Body/2014/onebody.pdf.

Knutson, Lebethe, et al. *Called Gathered Sent: A Bible Study Guide on the Role of Men and Women in Church and Society.* Cape Town: Evangelical Lutheran Church in Southern Africa (ELCSA), 2004.

Kuck, Mary Hills, ed. *Jamaica Praying: A Manual for HIV and AIDS Sensitive Liturgies and Sermons.* Kingston, Jamaica: United Theological College of the West Indies, 2014.

Kurian, Manoj. "An Ecumenical Framework for a Liberative Human Sexuality: Toward a Culture of Justice and Peace." *The Ecumenical Review* 64, no. 3 (October 2012): 338–45.

Longchar, A.Wati. *Health, Healing and Wholeness: Asian Theological Perspectives on HIV/AIDS.* Geneva: ETE-WCC/CAA, 2005.

Lubaale, Nicta. *Pastoral Action on HIV and AIDS: Training Guidelines on the Pastoral Aspects of the HIV Epidemic.* Called to Care series. Oxford: Strategies for Hope Trust, 2008.

_____. *Community Action on HIV and AIDS: Training Guidelines on Community Based Issues Related to HIV and AIDS*. Called to Care series. Oxford: Strategies for Hope Trust, 2008.

Lux, Steven, and Kristine Greenaway. *Scaling Up Effective Partnerships: A Guide to Working with Faith-based Organisations in the Response to HIV and AIDS*. Geneva: Ecumenical Advocacy Alliance, 2006. http://www.e-alliance.ch/en/s/hivaids/mobilizing-resources/faith-literacy/index.html.

Maldonado, Jorge E., ed. *A Guide to HIV/AIDS Pastoral Counselling*. Geneva: WCC Publications, 1990. http://www.wcc-coe.org/wcc/what/mission/guide.html.

Matthey, Jacques, ed. *Come Holy Spirit, Heal and Reconcile! Called in Christ to be Reconciling and Healing Communities*. Report of the WCC Conference on World Mission and Evangelism, Athens, Greece, 9–16 May 2005, Geneva: WCC Publications, 2008.

McGilvray, James C. *The Quest for Health and Wholeness*. Tübingen: German Institute for Medical Missions, 1981.

Mchombo, William, Joyce Larko Steiner, Dennis Milanzi, and Alfred Sebahene. *Call to Me: How the Bible Speaks in the Age of AIDS*. Called to Care series. Oxford: Strategies for Hope Trust, 2010.

Moyo, Fulata Lusungu. *Parenting: A Journey of Love: Knowledge and Skills for Parents and Guardians*. Called to Care series. Oxford: Strategies for Hope Trust, 2011.

Njoroge, Nyambura J., ed. "HIV: Ecumenical and Interfaith Responses." *The Ecumenical Review* 63, no. 4 (December 2011): 363–460.

Parry, Susan, *Beacons of Hope: HIV-Competent Churches—A Framework for Action*. Geneva: WCC Publications, 2008.

_____, ed. *Practicing Hope: A Handbook for Building HIV and AIDS Competence in the Churches*. EHAIA series. Geneva: WCC Publications, 2014.

Paterson, Gillian. *Whose Ministry? A Ministry of Healthcare for the Year 2000*. Risk Books. Geneva: WCC Publications, 1993.

_____. *Love in a Time of AIDS: Women, Health and the Challenge of HIV*. Risk Books. Geneva: WCC Publications,1996. Also published in the USA under the title *Women in the Time of AIDS*. Maryknoll, NY: Orbis, 1997.

_____. *AIDS-Related Stigma: Thinking Outside the Box—The Theological Challenge*. Geneva: EAA/WCC, 2005. http://www.e-alliance.ch/en/s/hivaids/stigma/aids-related-stigma-resource/index.html.

_____. "Escaping the Gender Trap: Unravelling Patriarchy in a Time of AIDS." In Regina Ammicht-Quinn and Hille Hacker, eds., *AIDS*, Concilium 2007/3. London: SCM Press, 2007.

_____, ed. *HIV Prevention: A Global Theological Conversation*. Geneva: Ecumenical Advocacy Alliance, 2009. http://www.e-alliance.ch/en/s/hivaids/publications/theological-conversation/index.html.

_____, and Callie Long, eds. *Dignity, Freedom, and Grace: Christian Perspectives on HIV, AIDS, and Human Rights*. Geneva: WCC Publications, 2016.

Prabhakar, Samson, and Mor Koorilos Geevarghese, eds. *HIV/AIDS: A Challenge to Theological Education*. Bangalore: BTESSC, SATHRI, 2004.

Rankin, Judy, Renate Cochrane, and the Khulakahle Child Counselling and Training Forum. *The Child Within: Connecting with Children Who Have Experienced Grief and Loss*. Called to Care series. Oxford: Strategies for Hope Trust, 2008.

Rubenson, Birgitta. *What Is AIDS? A Manual for Health Workers*. Geneva: WCC Publications, 1987.

_____. *Learning about HIV and AIDS: A Manual for Pastors and Teachers*. Geneva: WCC Publications, 1987, 1989; rev. eds.: 1994, 2002, 2006.

Russell, Letty R., ed. *The Church with AIDS: Renewal in the Midst of Crisis*. Louisville: Westminster John Knox, 1990.

Sander, Claudia, ed. *Neglected Dimensions in Health and Healing: Concepts and Explorations in an Ecumenical Perspective*. Study Document no. 3. Tübingen: DIFÄM, 2001.

Schuele, Elisabeth, and Astrid Berner-Rodoreda. *HIV & AIDS, Gender, and Domestic Violence Implications for Policy and Practice*. Dialogue no. 3. Stuttgart: Brot für die Welt/DIFÄM, 2010.

Sephuma, Thabo. *Discrimination, Isolation, Denial: A Resource and Action Guide on Travel Restrictions against People Living with HIV*. Geneva: Ecumenical Advocacy Alliance, 2008. http://www.e-alliance.ch/en/s/hivaids/publications/discrimination-isolation-denial/index.html.

Sheerattan-Bisnauth, Patricia, and Phillip Vinod Peacock. *Created in God's Image: From Hegemony to Partnership—A Church Manual on Men as Partners: Promoting Positive Masculinities*. Geneva: World Communion of Reformed Churches/World Council of Churches, 2010. http://menengage.org/resources/created-gods-image-hegemony-partnership-church-manual-men-partners-promoting-positive-masculinities/.

Skjelmerud, Anne, and Christopher Tusubira. *Confronting AIDS Together: Participatory Methods in Addressing the HIV/AIDS Epidemic: Including Learning from the WCC Experience in East and Central Africa*. Oslo/Geneva: Centre for Partnership Development, in collaboration with WCC, 1997.

Speicher, Sara, and Janice Wilson. *Exploring Solutions: How to Talk about HIV Prevention in the Church*. Geneva: Ecumenical Advocacy Alliance, 2007.

http://www.e-alliance.ch/en/s/hivaids/publications/exploring-solutions/index.html.

Steinitz, Lucy Y. *Making It Happen: A Guide to Help Your Congregation Do HIV/AIDS Work*. Called to Care series. Oxford: Strategies for Hope Trust, 2005.

_____, and Eunice Kamaara. *My Life—Starting Now: Knowledge and Skills for Young Adolescents*. Called to Care series. Oxford: Strategies for Hope Trust, 2010.

Tengatenga, James, and Anne Bayley. *Time to Talk: A Guide to Family Life in the Age of AIDS*. Called to Care series. Oxford: Strategies for Hope Trust, 2006.

Wilson, Pamela M. *Our Whole Lives (OWL): Sexuality Education Program Geared toward Youth in Grades 7 to 9*. Cleveland, OH: United Church of Christ Justice and Witness Ministries/Boston: Unitarian Universalist Association, 2007. http://www.uccresources.com/products/our-whole-lives-curriculum?variant=857888961.

United Church of Christ in the Philippines (UCCP). "Let Grace Be Total." United Church of Christ in the Philippines Statement on Lesbian, Gay, Bisexual, and Transgender (LGBT) Concerns—in response to the Churches' 2010 General Assembly request to come out with a Statement that addresses the issue of LGBT consistent with the theology and Statement of Faith of the UCCP. The Faith and Order Commission, 08 January 2014.

Vorster, J. M. "HIV/AIDS and Human Rights." *The Ecumenical Review* 55, no. 4 (October 2003): 345–61.

World Council of Churches (WCC). "The CMC Story 1968–1998." *Contact* 161/162 (1998).

_____. "Issue Focus—HIV & AIDS." *Ministerial Formation* 102 (January 2004)

_____. "List of Declarations and Policy Statements by Churches and Faith-based Organizations from 2001 to 2004." 2005.

_____. "Towards a Policy on HIV/AIDS in the Workplace: A Working Document." 2005.

_____. "AIDS: What Are the Churches Doing?" *Contact* 117 (December 1990). http://www.oikoumene.org/en/what-we-do/health-and-healing/117Dec1990AIDSWhatarethechurchesdoing.pdf.

_____. *The Vision and the Future of CMC: 25 Years of CMC*. Geneva: CMC—Churches Action for Health/WCC Publications, 1995.

_____. "Women and AIDS: Building Healing Communities." *Contact* 144 (August-September 1995). http://www.oikoumene.org/en/what-we-do/health-and-healing/144AugSept1995WomenandAIDSbuildinghealingcommunities.pdf.

_____. *Facing AIDS: The Challenge, the Churches' Response.* A WCC Study Document. Geneva: WCC Publications, 1997 (1st ed.). Reprinted in 2000, 2001, 2002 and 2004. http://wcc-coe.org/wcc/what/mission/ehaia-pdf/facing-aids-eng.pdf.

_____. "HIV & AIDS and Malaria." *Contact* 177/178 (January 2004). http://www.oikoumene.org/en/what-we-do/health-and-healing/con177178.pdf.

_____. "HIV Prevention: Current Issues and New Technologies." *Contact* 182 (August 2006). http://www.oikoumene.org/en/what-we-do/health-and-healing/con182.pdf.

_____. "HIV and AIDS Treatment: Faith-Based Organizations (FBOs) Get Involved." *Contact* 185 (October-December 2007). http://www.oikoumene.org/en/what-we-do/health-and-healing/con185_octdec_2007.pdf.

_____. "HIV and AIDS in the New Global Era: A Holistic Approach for Dignity of Life." *Contact* 194 (December 2013). http://www.oikoumene.org/en/what-we-do/health-and-healing/Contact194_EN.pdf.

Weinreich, Sonja, and Christopher Benn. *AIDS—Meeting the Challenge: Data, Facts, Background.* Geneva: WCC Publications, 2004. Trans. from German: *AIDS—Eine Krankheit verändert die Welt. Daten—Fakten—Hintergründe.* Frankfurt am Main: Verlag Otto Lembeck, 2003.

Wilkinson, John. *Christian Healing and the Congregation: The Healing Church.* World Council Studies no. 3. Geneva: WCC Publications, 1965.

West, Gerald, and Phumzile Zondi-Mabezela. "The Bible Story That Became a Campaign: The Tamar Campaign in South Africa (and Beyond)." *Ministerial Formation* 103 (July 2004): 12–14. http://ujamaa.ukzn.ac.za/Files/the bible story.pdf.

World Alliance of Reformed Churches. *Created in God's Image: From Hierarchy to Partnership. A Church Manual for Gender Awareness and Leadership Development.* Geneva: World Alliance of Reformed Churches, 2003.

World Vision. *Champions of Hope: A Collection of Short Stories.* Nairobi/Johannesburg/Dakar: World Vision International, 2009. http://wvi.org/sites/default/files/champions_of_hope_0.pdf.

World YWCA. "YWCA Safe Spaces for Women and Girls: A Global Model for Change, Mobilising Young Women Leadership on SRHR and HIV." 2014. http://www.worldywca.org/Resources/YWCA-Publications/YWCA-Safe-Spaces-for-Women-and-Girls-A-Global-Model-for-Change.

_____. *Reclaiming and Redefining Rights—ICPD+20: Status of Sexual and Reproductive Health and Rights in Africa.* Monitoring Report. Geneva: World YWCA, 2013. http://arrow.org.my/wp-content/uploads/2015/04/ICPD-20-Africa_Monitoring-Report_2013.pdf.

Other Journals and Publications

Atun, Rifat, et al. "Long-Term Financing Needs for HIV Control in Sub-Saharan Africa in 2015–2050: A Modelling Study." *BMJ Open* 6, no. 3 (6 March 2016). http://bmjopen.bmj.com/content/6/3/e009656.abstract.

Betron, Myra, Gary Barker, Juan Manuel Contreras, and Dean Peacock. *Men, Masculinities and HIV/AIDS: Strategies for Action*. Washington, DC: International Center for Research on Women/Rio de Janeiro: Instituto Promundo/Cape Town MenEngage Alliance and Sonke Gender Justice Network, 2008.

Burket, Mary K. *Advancing Reproductive Health and Family Planning through Religious Leaders and Faith-Based Organizations*. Pathfinder International. August 2006. http://www.pathfind.org/site/DocServer/FBO_final_reference.pdf?docID=6901.

Campbell, Catherine, Morten Skovdal, and Andrew Gibbs. "Creating Social Spaces to Tackle AIDS-Related Stigma: Reviewing the Role of Church Groups in Sub-Saharan Africa." *AIDS and Behaviour* 15, no. 6 (August 2011): 1204–19. http://uib.academia.edu/MortenSkovdal/Papers/199897/Creating_social_spaces_to_tackle_AIDS-related_stigma_Reviewing_the_role_of_Church_groups_in_sub-Saharan_Africa.

Cochrane, James R., Barbara Schmid, and T. Cutts, eds. *When Religion and Health Align: Mobilizing Religious Health Assets For Transformation*. Pietermaritzburg: Cluster Publications, 2011. http://www.religion.uct.ac.za/religion/staff/academicstaff/jamescochrane#sthash.cmQAgTnV.dpuf.

Denis, Philippe. *Never Too Small to Remember: Memory Work and Resilience in Times of AIDS*. Pietermaritzburg: Cluster Publications, 2005.

Dimmock, Franck, Jill Olivier, and Quentin Wodon. *Half a Century Young: The Christian Health Associations in Africa*. MPRA Paper no. 45369 (March 2013). http://mpra.ub.uni-muenchen.de/45369/. *See esp. the "Overview on history, members, and main activities of the Christian Health Associations.*

Dube, Musa W. *The HIV and AIDS Bible: Selected Essays*. Scranton, PA: University of Scranton Press, 2008.

———. "On Being Firefighters: Curriculum Transformation in the HIV & AIDS Context." *Studia Historiae Ecclesiasticae* 35–Supplement (December 2009).

———. "Mainstreaming HIV/AIDS in African Religious and Theological Studies." In Afe Adogame, Ezra Chitando, and Bolaji Bateye, eds., *African Traditions in the Study of Religion in Africa*, 77–95. New York/London: Routledge, 2012.

————, and Tinyiko S. Maluleke, eds. *Missionalia: Southern Africa Journal of Missiology* 29, no. 2 (August 2001): passim.

————, and Musimbi Kanyoro. *Grant Me Justice! HIV/AIDS and Gender Readings of the Bible.* Pietermaritzburg: Cluster Publications, 2004.

Georgetown University—Berkley Centre for Religion, Peace, and World Affairs. "A Discussion with Rev. Canon Gideon Byamugisha." 3 May 2009. http://berkleycenter.georgetown.edu/interviews/a-discussion-with-rev-canon-gideon-byamugisha-founder-african-network-of-religious-leaders-living-with-or-personally-affected-by-hiv-aids.

Grundmann, Christoffer H. *Gesandt zu heilen. Aufkommen und Entwicklung der Ärztlichen Mission im neunzehnten Jahrhundert.* Missionswissenschaftliche Forschungen Bd. 12. Gütersloh: Gutersloher Verlaugshaus G. Mohn, 1992.

Gunner. Göran, ed. *Vulnerability, Churches, and HIV.* Church of Sweden, Research Series 1. Portland, OR: Pickwick, 2009.

Haddad, Beverley. "'We Pray but We Cannot Heal': Theological Challenges Posed by the HIV/AIDS Crisis." *Journal of Theology for South Africa* 125 (2006): 80–90.

Hallman, D. G., ed. *AIDS Issues: Confronting the Challenge.* New York: Pilgrim, 1989.

Litsios, Socrates. "The Christian Medical Commission and the Development of WHO's Primary Health Care Approach." *American Journal of Public Health* 94, no. 11 (November 2004): 1884–93. http://www.ncbi.nlm.nih.gov/pmc/articles/PMC1448555/.

Njoroge, Nyambura J., and Musa W. Dube. *Talitha Cum! Theologies of African Women.* Pietermaritzburg: Cluster Publications, 2001.

McNeill, Donald P., Douglas A. Morrison, and Henri J. M. Nouwen. *Compassion: A Reflection on the Christian Life.* New York: Doubleday/Image Books, 1982.

Olivier, Jill, James R. Cochrane, Barbara Schmid, and Lauren Graham. *ARHAP Bibliography: Working in a Bounded Field of Unknowing.* Cape Town: African Religious Health Assets Programme, 2006.

————, Gary S. D. Leonard, and Barbara Schmid. *The Cartography of HIV and AIDS: A Partially Annotated Bibliography.* The Collaborative for HIV and AIDS, Religion and Theology (CHART)— An Initiative of the School of Religion and Theology, University of KwaZulu-Natal. January 2012. http://www.cabsa.org.za/sites/default/files/CHART_VI_bibliog_Jan2012.pdf.

PEPFAR. *A Firm Foundation: The PEPFAR Consultation on the Role of Faith-based Organizations in Sustaining Community and Country Leadership in the*

Response to HIV/AIDS. Washington, DC: U.S. Department of State, 2012. http://www.pepfar.gov/documents/organization/195614.pdf.

Phiri, Isabel Apawo, Beverley Haddad, Madipoane Masenya, and Ngwana Mphahlele. *African Women, HIV/AIDS, and Faith Communities*. Pietermaritzburg: Cluster Publications, 2003.

Van Klinken, Adriaan, and Ezra Chitando. "Masculinities, HIV and Religion in Africa." In Emma Tomalin, ed., *The Routledge Handbook of Religions and Global Development*, 127–37. New York and London: Routledge, 2015.

Welch Kline, Rebecca J., and Nelya J. McKenzie. "HIV/AIDS, Women, and Threads of Discrimination: Tapestry of Disenfranchisement." In Eileen Berlin Ray, ed., *Communication and Disenfranchisement: Social Health Issues and Implications*, 365–86. Mahwah, NJ: Routledge, 1996.

WHO

Karpf, Ted, and Alex Ross, eds. *Building from Common Foundations: The World Health Organization and Faith-Based Organizations in Primary Healthcare*. Geneva: World Health Organization, 2008. http://apps.who.int/iris/bitstream/10665/43884/1/9789241596626_eng.pdf.

UNAIDS

Sidibé Michel, *Churches: Barricades against Exclusion*, UNAIDS Executive Director's address to the 10th Assembly of the World Council of Churches, 31 October 2013 Busan, Republic of Korea. http://www.unaids.org/sites/default/files/sub_landing/files/20131031_EXD_SP_WCC_en.pdf.

UNAIDS. *A Report of a Theological Workshop Focusing on HIV- and AIDS-related Stigma*. Windhoek, Namibia, 8 to 11 December 2003. Geneva: UNAIDS, 2004. http://data.unaids.org/Publications/IRC-pub06/jc1056_theological-report_en.pdf.

_____. *The GAP Report*. Geneva: UNAIDS, 2014. http://www.unaids.org/sites/default/files/media_asset/UNAIDS_Gap_report_en.pdf.

_____. "Fast-Track: Ending the AIDS Epidemic by 2030. 2014. http://www.unaids.org/en/resources/documents/2014/JC2686_WAD2014report.

_____. *On the Fast-Track to End AIDS by 2030: Focus on Location and Population*. Geneva: UNAIDS, 2015. http://www.unaids.org/sites/default/files/media_asset/WAD2015_report_en_part01.pdf.